FURTHER RESEARCH FOR

CW01084773

Education for Care Series

Further Research for Nursing
A New Guide for the Enquiring Nurse

Edited by

JILL MACLEOD CLARK PhD, BSc, SRN

and

LISBETH HOCKEY OBE, PhD, BSc, SRN, SCM, QN,
HVCert, RNT, FRCN

With 11 contributors

Scutari Press

London

© Scutari Press 1989
A division of Scutari Projects Ltd, the publishing company of
the Royal College of Nursing

First published 1989
Reprinted 1991, 1992

British Library Cataloguing in Publication Data

Further research for nursing.
  1. Medicine. Nursing. Research
  I. Clark, Jill Macleod   II. Hockey,
  Lisbeth
  610.73'072

ISBN 1 871364 14 0

Printed and bound in Great Britain by
Biddles Ltd, Guildford and King's Lynn

Contributors

JULIA I BROOKING *Senior Lecturer in Psychiatric Nursing, Institute of Psychiatry, University of London*

JILL MACLEOD CLARK *Senior Lecturer, Department of Nursing Studies, King's College, University of London*

PHILIP DARBYSHIRE *Research Student, Nursing Research Unit, Department of Nursing Studies, University of Edinburgh*

PAULINE FIELDING *Chief Nursing Officer, Whipps Cross Hospital, London*

JULIET HAWKES *Clinical Outcomes Programme Co-ordinator, Wessex Regional Health Authority*

ROSAMUND HERBERT *Lecturer, Department of Nursing Studies, King's College, University of London*

LISBETH HOCKEY OBE *Formerly Director, Nursing Research Unit, Department of Nursing Studies, University of Edinburgh*

JENNIFER M HUNT *Nursing Officer, Department of Health and Social Services, London*

JENNIFER LITTLEWOOD *Senior Lecturer, Nursing and Community Health Studies, Centre for the Study of Primary Care, North East Thames RHA, London*

PETER LOWTHIAN *Clinical Nurse Specialist, Royal National Orthopaedic Hospital, London*

v

DONNA M MEAD *Senior Lecturer, Department of Nursing, North East Wales Institute of Further Education, Wrexham*

TRICIA MURPHY-BLACK *Midwife Research Officer, Nursing Research Unit, Department of Nursing Studies, University of Edinburgh*

JENIFER WILSON-BARNETT *Professor and Head of the Department of Nursing Studies, King's College, University of London*

Contents

Preface

Further Research for Nursing is a 'new generation' book which
has been designed and written to help today's nurses to accept
and appreciate the role of research in their work. We have
retained a similar format to that used in this book's predecessor
and companion volume – *Research for Nursing* – as our readers
have told us they found it helpful. However, the contents of
this new volume comprise largely up-dated material and will
thus, it is hoped, complement the original book.

Nurses have seen many changes in their profession since
1979, although one thing has *not* changed. That is the need for
every nurse to become more aware of the importance of
research and to recognise the actual and potential contribution
that research can make to all areas of nursing, midwifery and
health visiting. Many official reports, including Project 2000,
the British nursing profession's blueprint for the next century,
continue to stress the need for research, and the case for developing a research base for professional practice has become
stronger than ever.

One of the main functions of this book is to help nurses to
incorporate a knowledge and understanding of research into
their work. This is achieved, we hope, by taking the reader on a
guided tour of recent and readily accessible research on various
topics. As a general principle we have tried to ensure that, as
far as possible, the research material included is:

1. relevant to British nursing, midwifery or health visiting;
2. readily available and as recent as possible;
3. illustrative of a range of research techniques and methods.

Just occasionally, we have found it necessary to refer to
unpublished work, usually in the form of a university thesis.

This has been done where the research seemed relevant but where no published version of it was available at the time of going to press.

It is now ten years since the publication of the companion volume, *Research for Nursing*. During that time there has been a proliferation of specialised research literature and a rapid growth of knowledge in many aspects of nursing. For this reason, we have not attempted to review this recent literature ourselves but have asked a group of experts to provide a succinct overview of recent research in their own field.

The book is divided into three main parts. In Part I an attempt is made to introduce research in a straightforward way by discussing its meaning, its relevance to nursing and some methodological as well as ethical principles. At the end of this section, readers will find a glossary of commonly-used research terms. Parts II and III of the book contain the overviews of research in 12 different areas or topics.

In each of the chapters in Part II, research which illuminates the nursing care of specific groups of patients or clients is explored. In Part III the focus moves to a number of more general nursing issues, such as pressure area care, the role of clinical observations and manpower planning, which have been examined through the medium of research.

Each chapter author has presented a broad overview of the research material and also included a précis of one or two specific studies. As in *Research for Nursing*, this approach is designed to help nurses to become more familiar with the stages of the research process and to illustrate some of the different methods used to tackle research questions. The book concludes with a chapter which glimpses into the future and examines the role of research as a change agent.

The omission of an index is deliberate, as both technical research terms and different aspects and areas of nursing research tend to be better understood in context. Hopefully readers will find the whole book irresistible, but we have attempted to meet the needs of those who wish to be selective by ensuring that each chapter is carefully structured and relatively short.

It is important to make it clear that while the aim of this book is to increase the reader's understanding of research techniques, particularly as they apply to specific research questions, it is not intended to be a text on research methodology or a critical review of completed research. Many helpful texts covering these issues are now available and a selection of them is listed on page 26. We should also emphasise that almost all research has deficiencies and it is beyond the scope of this book to discuss the merits or otherwise of any given piece of work.

We hope that this book, reinforced by the original research reports quoted, will help to stimulate practising nurses to use available research with greater eagerness and understanding. We also hope that it will help them to develop their skills of enquiry and, in consequence, raise new research questions. Conversely, we hope that nurse researchers, in partnership with practising nurses, will take up some of the many nursing problems which are, as yet, devoid of a scientifically credible knowledge base. The challenges to practising nurses and researchers abound.

This book could not have been written without the existence of the many research reports and studies described in the text. We would like to acknowledge the co-operation of the authors concerned and express our gratitude to all our friends, colleagues and fellow researchers for their enthusiasm, support and contribution. We would also like to thank Patrick West for his continued encouragement and Joan Armstrong for so expertly typing the manuscript.

Jill Macleod Clark
Lisbeth Hockey

1989

Part I: Understanding Research

Introduction

JILL MACLEOD CLARK and LISBETH HOCKEY

The purpose of this book is to demonstrate to all nurses,* regardless of level or specialty, that research is relevant to their work. In order to understand the contribution that research can make to nursing we strongly recommend reading the first two chapters before 'dipping into' chapters in Part II which may seem more alluring!

In the first chapter the basic principles of a research approach are outlined to show how this approach differs from common-sense reasoning or 'experience'. We attempt to address the issue of why nurses should be concerned about and involved in research. We also suggest that all nurses should ask critical questions about the way that research is undertaken, the resources it uses and the way in which research findings are implemented. Research raises important ethical issues of which all nurses should be aware and some of the most important of these are outlined in the last section of Chapter 1.

In the second chapter we have set ourselves the almost impossible task of giving a simple overview of research design and method. The reader must appreciate that the presentation is grossly oversimplified. Our aim is to help nurses in their reading and understanding of the studies referred to in the other parts of the book. Each of these studies has its own research design and method, and different methods produce different kinds of findings. In the interpretation of research findings, the method used to produce them should be understood. An analogy from nursing might clarify this point. A

*For the sake of simplicity the female gender has been used for 'nurse' throughout the book.

1

patient's body temperature may be taken orally or rectally; in the interpretation of the readings it is important to know which method was used.

Because the process of research has its own principles and techniques it also has a language of its own. Some technical terminology is necessary to describe and to understand research and we have included in a glossary a few terms commonly used in research in the hope that some of the mystique of unfamiliar words might be removed.

In the use of this book, we suggest that when reading about some of the studies, where the research design and method are described, the information given in Part I should be used for reference purposes. In this way, a measure of understanding of research will be acquired in the easiest and most stimulating way.

Chapter 1

The Relevance of Research to Nursing

JILL MACLEOD CLARK and LISBETH HOCKEY

In our earlier volume, we stated that nursing research was a relatively 'new' discipline. That was 10 years ago, so it can no longer be called 'new'. There has certainly been a remarkable increase in research endeavour and also a more consistent inclusion of research in basic nursing curricula during the last decade. There has also been some general increase in research interest in the profession. However, it is not possible to make quite such a positive statement about the implementation and appropriate use of research findings among practitioners in nursing, midwifery and health visiting.

Many highly experienced nurses still appear to feel that their practice, based on rich experience, requires little or no change. It seems to work well and no-one is complaining. They wonder what 'all the fuss is about'. Their point of view deserves to be taken seriously and it would be misguided to disregard the contribution that experience has made to the growth of knowledge. It is important, however, to understand the difference between subjectively accumulated, intuitive knowledge and the type of knowledge which is generated by scientifically credible methods. The two approaches to the building up of knowledge are not mutually exclusive; in fact, they are interrelated. The experience of nurses is essential to the further development of nursing.

There is no doubt that nursing and research need each other, and this volume is intended to strengthen the bridges between them.

The meaning of research

So, what is research and what has it to offer?

First, it must be recognised that research in nursing is fundamentally no different from research in any field. There is no shortage of definitions, ranging from the over-simplified to the over-obtuse. For the purpose of this book, we broadly adhere to the definition used in the previous edition:

> Research is an attempt to increase available knowledge by the discovery of new facts or relationships through systematic enquiry.

Not all research achieves an increase in the knowledge base of a discipline. However, provided that the enquiry follows systematic principles, it still qualifies for the status of research. Thus, it is the method of the enquiry which is the decisive factor. Systematic enquiry must follow certain basic steps; the sequence of these steps is known as the research process. The enquiring nurse will discern the analogy between nursing and research in terms of a definable process. Both the nursing process (or the process of nursing) and the research process consist of a sequence of systematic steps. Also, just as the process of nursing may be guided by a variety of models or conceptual frameworks, so can the research process adopt different strategies largely depending on the initial question being asked. It is for this reason that we asked our group of experts to give an outline of one or two studies, using the basic format of the main research question, the appropriate research design and method, the main findings and some implications for nursing. A brief overview of some general research approaches including basic steps in the research process is presented in Chapter 2.

Having defined 'research', it remains to agree, at least for the purpose of this book, on the meaning of 'nursing research'. We like to think that any activity for which a nurse, midwife or health visitor is predominantly and appropriately responsible should be scientifically defensible. This presupposes that it should be exposed to research or nursing research. Clearly, this wide definition implies that the activities of teachers and administrators of nursing as well as those of clinically involved nurses require scientific study. Therefore, we would include research in nursing education and in nursing administration under the umbrella of 'nursing research'. As explained in the preface, however, we have slanted this volume towards clinical nursing research, mainly because we believe that it is in this area that the bridges between nursing and research require urgent reinforcement.

The need for and relevance of nursing research

The need for research is prompted by three main developments in nursing. In the first place, there is increasing pressure on nurses to defend their activities in terms of resource use. There is a widespread quest for quality measures in many disciplines and nursing is no exception. In the UK, where attempts are being made to run the National Health Service on principles taken from industrial management, such a quest is challenging the nursing profession in an unprecedented manner. Secondly, intelligent entrants into the nursing profession are now more likely than ever to demand acceptable reasons for the procedures they are being taught. Long-standing tradition or local convention is not likely to pacify, indeed, should not pacify the enquiring nurse. Thirdly, progress in the academic education of nurses and in the professionalisation of nursing gives a necessary and desirable impetus to research awareness and research pursuit.

As far as the relevance of research is concerned, it is necessary to acknowledge that the discipline is amenable to research and that it is possible for nurses to use research findings as a basis for practice. Some research may merely help nurses towards a better understanding of certain aspects of nursing, without necessarily changing practice. For example, knowledge of the 'dying' process, as identified and described in the classic study by Kübler Ross (1973), can help a nurse or other caring person to understand and thus be supportive of a dying patient's anger or despair. The relevance of such research can hardly be disputed. The stimulation and excitement of research are also important. It is clearly beneficial to any workers in whatever sphere to find their work stimulating and exciting, and nurses are being increasingly encouraged to be involved in both research and practice.

There are those nurses who consider that research is reserved for an academic elite and there are those nurse researchers who prefer to be divorced from the practice of nursing. They must be reminded that most applied research begins with an astute observation in the respective area: 'Why is it that . . .?' 'Could there be a better way of doing . . .?' 'What is the purpose of . . .?' 'Could it be omitted from the daily routine?' etc. The initial observation and question arising from the real-world situation are crucial to the development and potential usefulness of any research project. We must, therefore, foster the essential interrelationship between nursing practice and nursing research.

Developments in nursing research

After relatively slow beginnings in the field of nursing research in the UK in the late 1950s and early 1960s, progress has been encouragingly rapid. The main reasons for this upsurge lie, undoubtedly, in the wider educational opportunities for nurses and in the increasing acknowledgement of the need for nursing research by administrators at all levels, from government departments to clinical areas.

Until 20 years ago, nurses were largely dependent on members of other disciplines, especially the social scientists, for the study of their own profession. Thus, sociologists and psychologists have made a substantial contribution to the literature of nursing research, and this may explain the early emphasis on studies of nurses rather than of nursing. Many of the research techniques now used by nurses have their origin in the social sciences. The biological sciences clearly have a great deal to offer and a few nurses have applied physiological measures in their studies of nursing.

It is reasonable to assume that nursing research will increase in importance. Educational reform, as envisaged in Project 2000 (UKCC 1986), is bound to encourage a spirit of enquiry and stimulate research-based teaching. Administrative changes in the National Health Service, with their increasing emphasis on cost containment and demonstrable measures of effectiveness and efficiency, are bound to evoke research responses. Evidence can only be provided by research, whether this lies in the systematic study of existing statistical data or in the generation of new, purpose-designed projects. In nursing practice, the call for high standards of care must result in increasing attempts to develop scientifically credible indicators of quality. Our American colleagues have led the way in this particular area of research as discussed in Chapter 14. Studies of the use of manpower and appropriate skill mix are inherent in such work. In general, the climate for the pursuit of nursing research is not only favourable but compelling. It is now incumbent on the British nursing profession to build on and refine existing knowledge and techniques.

Ethical issues

A commitment to research at whatever level raises a number of ethical issues. In the first place it must be taken seriously as an integral part of professional responsibility. To pay lip service to research is to contradict the principles of professionalism. It is a pretence which is not merely dishonest but may even be harmful by offending the code of conduct to which a nurse should pledge herself. The general public who entrust their care to nurses as professionals have a right to expect adherence to a recognised code of conduct. An obvious and essential part of such a code of conduct is a serious and honest shouldering of professional responsibility.

Research must be seen as a team activity. It involves all groups of nurses, not only those with a specific research responsibility. Practising nurses must continue in the spirit of research mindedness engendered during their professional preparation; they must question accepted practices. Administrators in the clinical areas must respond positively to such questions. They must also facilitate the appropriate conduct of research in their area. Researchers must gain competence, finance and access. All nurses must be willing to read available research reports, attempt to understand them and be willing to make appropriate use of the findings. All these activities have ethical implications.

A serious commitment to research does not imply an unquestioning acceptance of research activity or of research findings. Research as an activity, just as nursing as an activity, has its own ethical code of practice which must be observed by the researcher. The reader is referred to *Ethics Related to Research in Nursing* (RCN 1977) which provides a helpful summary of the ethical issues involved in research. Just as the general public have a right to expect a recognised code of conduct from the professional nurse, so the nurse has a right to expect a recognised code of conduct from a researcher who wishes to undertake research in the area for which she is responsible. The nurse should have a knowledge of the code of conduct to be expected from a researcher, for without such knowledge she is unable to assure herself that it is observed. The main points on which a nurse giving access to a researcher should assure herself are:

1. The aims and purpose of the research.
2. That there are no unnecessary risks or inconveniences to patients or staff.
3. That respect for confidentiality and anonymity is maintained as appropriate.
4. The competence of the researcher.
5. The intended use of research findings.

Although a newly qualified nurse will not usually be called upon to provide access to an area for research purposes, she is entitled to information on the above points. It is part of the research code of ethics to explain the research to all the people involved in it and to provide the requested information.

Aims and purpose of research Our definition of research (given on page 4) implies that all research attempts to increase available knowledge; if it fails to make such an attempt, it does not qualify as research. Therefore, all research has a potential for good, as an increase of knowledge can only be beneficial. It is possible, however, that the new knowledge sought by the researcher is not seen to have a direct application to nursing; it may be a quest for satisfaction of a purely academic curiosity. Such research tends to be referred to as 'pure' (Notter 1974) whereas research undertaken with the specific aim of applying the findings would be referred to as 'applied' research. The distinction, though important, is not always clear cut. Some 'pure' research is later seen to have a direct and practical application to nursing, while some 'applied' research may be found to be of academic value only. Therefore, permission to undertake research should not be made dependent on its immediate potential for application. Some research, however, has unrealistic aims and the researcher may justifiably be asked to re-define them.

Nurses who are asked to help with research, either by answering questions or by allowing themselves to be observed, should be given the option to refuse. A commitment to research implies, however, that the reasons for refusal should be based on something more concrete than mere apathy and also that they are divulged to the researcher. For example, there is no shame in not wishing to answer questions on perceived needs of dying patients when one has recently been bereaved. There may be many other perfectly understandable reasons for not wishing to be involved in a specific research project and it helps the researcher and the value of the research if these reasons are known.

Risks or inconveniences to patients or staff Some research attempts to compare different methods of giving care, and necessitates one group of patients being subjected to a form of care which may be thought by some to carry certain risks or to deprive the patients of certain known or expected benefits. For example, if a researcher wished to compare a new dressing technique with one which has stood the test of time, there may be an understandable reservation and diffidence in the first instance. The nurse giving consent to the research would expect reasonable assurance on the safety of the proposed technique, well confirmed by factual evidence, probably obtained under laboratory conditions. Sometimes, a certain amount of risk taking is inevitable, as the proposed research may be the only way of testing a new method of treatment. In such cases, provision for the safety of the patient must be built into the study design through frequent monitoring of the patient's condition, as should the right to discontinue the experimental procedure or treatment should undesirable symptoms occur.

Inconvenience to patients may be caused by asking them questions or by observing them. In all cases where patients are involved in the research their informed consent to what is proposed must be sought. Informed consent means that the patients agree to the study after having it explained to them as fully as possible. Any proposals for research involving patients or clients within the structure of the National Health Service have to be approved by a special committee to ensure the safeguarding of the patients' rights and safety.

Inconvenience to staff may be caused by disrupting their routine, by encroaching on time, by causing a feeling of threat. It is part of the ethical code of conduct for research that any such inconvenience should be reduced to an absolute minimum, if it cannot be prevented altogether. Most textbooks on research methods will include detailed advice to the researcher on how to achieve a relaxed and receptive research setting. For the purpose of this book's objective it is sufficient to say that the nurse at the receiving end of research, be it as the person giving permission, as a respondent or observed subject or as a user of the completed research, should assure herself that the research has, or had, a concern for the staff involved. The results of research in which the staff felt ill at ease, pressurised or unduly inconvenienced may have an undesirable bias.

Respect for confidentiality and anonymity   An important part of the code of ethics for researchers is to safeguard the confidentiality of information which has been collected as part of the research. Data made available for research purposes should not be passed on for any other purpose without the explicit permission of the person who has provided them either in a verbal response or by allowing himself to be observed. Anonymity, if promised, must be respected not only in the letter but also in the spirit. Thus, although a research report may not include any names, people described in it may be identifiable by virtue of their position. If this is a distinct possibility and the singling out of a particular individual cannot be avoided, his permission to publish the findings relevant to him must be sought. Sometimes the problem of identification is not related to people, but to geographical areas or to institutions. Some of the problems related to confidentiality and anonymity are described by Hockey (1985).

Competence of the researcher   Just as a nurse should not carry out a task for which she is not competent, at least not without adequate supervision, so a researcher should work within limits of competence. Often researchers apply a specific science to nursing research and it is important that they understand this science. An example would be the use of a psychological test as a means of collecting specific information.

In most instances, the researcher's competence is assured by the fact that funding for the study was obtained. Funding bodies take considerable care in ensuring that the research will be carried out, or at least supervised, by a competent person.

Research is costly, both in time and money. It may make demands on many people and should, therefore, be carried out with the greatest possible care and efficiency.

Intended use of research findings   Research findings should be used for the purpose stated by the researcher in the first instance, when permission to undertake the research is given. Research findings should be published and not suppressed. The way in which they are presented is an important part of research expertise, as inappropriate presentation may mislead the reader.

As this book is written specifically for the reader and potential user of research, it is emphasised that a careful reader should keep a watchful eye on the ethical issues alluded to. Where concern about offence of the ethical code of research is felt, it should be communicated to the author of the research publication in a constructive manner. Informed comment on published material is a professional responsibility. Some research findings have implications for wider implementation. It is also a professional responsibility to use such findings and to disseminate them as widely as possible.

References

Hockey L. (1985) *Nursing Research – Mistakes and Misconceptions*. Edinburgh: Churchill Livingstone

Kübler Ross E. (1973) *On Death and Dying*. London: Tavistock Publications

Notter L.E. (1974) *Essentials of Nursing Research*. New York: Springer-Verlag

RCN (1977) *Ethics Related to Research in Nursing*. London: Royal College of Nursing

United Kingdom Central Council for Nursing, Midwifery and Health Visiting (1986) *Project 2000*. London: UKCC

Chapter 2

Research Approaches and Methods – An Overview

JILL MACLEOD CLARK and LISBETH HOCKEY

There are various ways in which research approaches can and have been classified and most textbooks on research methodology include complex and sophisticated expositions. This chapter is intended to be a brief overview of the major approaches, designs and methods and is of necessity an over-simplification. A good proportion of nursing research to date has been empirical in approach, that is, the researcher collected information from the 'real' world by a variety of methods which are discussed later in this chapter. It is possible, however, to adopt an historical, a philosophical or a theoretical perspective.

Historical research

Historical research is important in terms of its potential to increase knowledge and understanding. In this type of research, documents and reports are analysed by the researcher who relates them to selected events, to developments or to the lives of individuals who are considered to have had an impact on the course of such developments and events. Ideally, the historical researcher will use primary sources of information, that is the original relevant document, such as an Act of Parliament, or a parliamentary question recorded in Hansard, rather than a comment on these. For example, a future nurse researcher may wish to study the development of nursing education in the UK. It would be advisable, among other possibilities, to consult the Nurses' Acts and the Report of the Committee and Commissions on Nursing, such as the Judge Report (RCN 1985), and the Cumberlege Report (DHSS 1986), in their original form. There are also many summaries of these documents, which are called secondary sources. Mostly, it is appropriate to undertake a thorough study of primary as well as secondary sources because comments on, and summaries of, the original documents may have influenced the course of events under the study.

Examples of historical research undertaken by nurses are studies by Davies (1980) and Maggs (1981). Each study was generated by specific questions, which is the common denominator for all research, but the frame of reference or starting point differed. The first study centred around the development of nursing education, while in the second study the focus of the research was on the influence of social control mechanisms in nursing. In each case the researcher made a thorough analysis of relevant events over a period of time, which in turn provided insights into our understanding of the present situation.

Philosophical research

Philosophical research uses the tools of logic and reason in an attempt to extend knowledge. It analyses words and their meaning, their use and their effect. It examines concepts, ideas and values which form a considerable part of our communication systems and our professional education and practice. The relevance of such research to a clearer understanding of nursing can easily be seen. We tend to use the term 'philosophical' rather too freely; philosophical research applies the academic discipline of philosophy to the research. To date, few nurses with this particular approach to research have emerged, at least in the UK. We would have preferred to use more recent literature as examples. Beginnings in philosophical research were made by Williams (1974) in a paper *Ideologies of Nursing: their meanings and implications*. Another British nurse researcher with a philosophical approach is Schröck who, in a paper concerned with aspects of health visiting, describes some of the issues which are the proper concern of the philosophical perspective (Schröck 1977). The work of Inman (1975), *Towards a Theory of Nursing Care*, also belongs to the category of philosophical research. Some of this work consists of a summary and synthesis of the 12 clinical studies undertaken under the auspices of the Royal College of Nursing as part of the overall Study of Nursing Care. Another part of the book deals with philosophical considerations. In an attempt to answer the question 'Is it possible to develop measures of the quality of care?', Inman invokes the theories of some influential philosophers. Concepts such as 'quality of nursing care' and 'needs of patients' are analysed and discussed. She contends that the quality of nursing care will only become amenable to measurement within the framework of a 'context–process–product model' and suggests how such a model might be created and empirically tested. Recommendations for further research are also made. Inman's work draws attention to the need for a closer examination of concepts used in nursing. She developed a classification system for the studies undertaken within the nursing care project in an attempt to relate their total contribution to the knowledge base of nursing.

A further example of the philosophical approach to research was undertaken in the USA by Smith (1981), who investigated a central concept in nursing – that of 'health'.

Theoretical research

The approach which distinguishes theoretical research in nursing from other types is its starting point from theories developed in any discipline and the application of these theories to the academic study of nursing without intervening empirical work. It may, however, lead to empirical work. An example of this type of research is *The Proper Study of the Nurse* (McFarlane 1970). In this research the underlying question was 'How can one study nursing in a scientific manner?'. A systems approach is suggested and examples of different systems are described; the researcher produced a theoretical framework within which studies of nursing might be undertaken. The theoretical exposition on the nature of criteria and the extensive bibliography are important parts of this contribution to nursing knowledge.

In recent years a great deal of energy has been devoted to the development of nursing theory, particularly in the USA. As a consequence, more researchers are attempting to integrate nursing theory into their work. The ultimate test of a theory is its predictive and explanatory power and we can perhaps expect to see a growth in explicit theory testing and deductive research in nursing during the next decade.

Theoretical research is often contrasted with practical research but this is a misuse of the term. Theoretical research has considerable practical potential and it may be more accurate to contrast it with empirical research.

Empirical research

There are two main approaches to the collection of data from people in real-life situations. Deductive research takes a given conceptual framework or theory as a starting point and the research project is designed to test this. Inductive research works in the opposite direction: the researcher begins the process with systematic observation of a given phenomenon or set of phenomena with the intention of developing a theory which can later be tested.

The deductive researcher relies on quantitative material and collects and tests data from a certain sample or a population. The qualitative researcher often works with small numbers, sometimes even single 'cases' or situations. The quantitative researcher collects the data in a standardised manner so that the results can be counted or quantified. The qualitative researcher allows the data collection to be guided by the actual individual situation; there is usually no attempt to quantify the results, although some structure is often imposed. The aim is, rather, to probe more deeply into the given situation and to reach quality in understanding.

Regrettably, a competitive divisive schism appears to have developed between the protagonists of the two approaches. Like most experienced qualitative researchers, such as Melia (1982) and Field and Morse (1985), we consider that both approaches have their rightful place in the development of nursing knowledge. They are not mutually exclusive. On the contrary, they can support each other. It is true that qualitative research findings cannot be generalised, but their potential for the insightful understanding of given situations is usually greater than that obtained from quantitative data, however large the sample. The two approaches serve different purposes and, providing they are pursued in scientifically acknowledged ways, following given ground rules and principles, they are both scientifically credible. Often, qualitative work is undertaken as a precursor to a quantitative study, as a means to explore the real situation and help the formulation of a testable hypothesis or a researchable question. Though useful for this purpose, its scope is much wider. For a helpful text on qualitative research design, the reader is referred to Field and Morse (1985).

Many different research designs or approaches are appropriate to the investigation of nursing and these include descriptive research, experimental research and action research.

Descriptive research   Descriptive research, as the term implies, describes a situation, using a scientific method for the purpose. The science lies in the precise definition of the terms used, in accurate documentation and precise measurements, where appropriate. It also implies adherence to the systematic steps of the research process, the principles of which are relevant to all research, whatever the approach taken.

Descriptive research design can take many different forms, only some of which are mentioned in this chapter. In the first place a distinction must be made between a survey approach and a case study approach.

A survey normally covers a large number of subjects in the enquiry, in an attempt to describe a situation which may have relevance elsewhere. Most surveys are designed on the basis of representative samples, which enables the researcher to claim application of his or her findings from a sample to a wider population within a calculable margin of error. For example, in the study of the role of the midwife undertaken by Robinson *et al.* (1983), data were collected from a sample of 4248 midwives who were working in 60 different health districts. A sample of this size is obviously more likely to produce data representative of midwives in general than a sample taken, say, from just one or two health districts.

In contrast to this, in case study research, information is obtained in depth from the detailed examination of one or very few subjects. Case studies can produce important findings for nursing and some nursing problems are especially suited to a case study approach rather than a survey approach. For example, Janes (1984) described her perceptions of nursing and nursing care from a participation observation study of one ward.

Another important distinction which needs to be made relates to the time scale of descriptive research projects. The time period of a survey is determined and no attempt is made to record any progress or change in the situation; the time period is taken as being fixed. For example, Beail (1985) spent many days in wards in order to be able to describe the 'current' situation in terms of interactions between nurses and mentally handicapped children. However, the researcher should always ensure that the period of time selected for study is not atypical. For this reason it is occasionally necessary that the data collection process takes place over a period of time in order to obtain the full picture of events. Such an extended period is particularly necessary when there is a known fluctuation of events, as, for example, in a week on a surgical ward which has two operation days within it.

In contrast to this prescribed time scale, there are other studies in which an attempt is made to describe how a situation and/or subjects change over a given period of time. The emphasis here is on the change. In a study of this kind, it is possible to take the current situation as a starting point and relate it to the time period preceding it; it would then be a retrospective study. For example, if one wished to study patterns of the length of in-patient stay, one could compare the current length of stay with past records in order to identify changes over time. However, in research which attempts to describe changes over time, the prospective approach is more common. Here, the researcher may follow his subjects, referred to as a cohort, through a given period of time, usually a circumscribed experience such as nurse training. Howard and Brooking (1987) followed this approach in their study of career patterns of undergraduate nurses.

Occasionally, time constraints or other reasons make a true longitudinal study impossible. Thus, if a researcher has only 3 years in which to undertake the work, it is impossible to follow student nurses through the whole of their 3-year training period; it would not leave time at the beginning for the preliminary work and the pilot study and it would leave no time to analyse the information and write the report. A special adaptation of the true longitudinal design is a cross-sectional longitudinal study. The difference here is that the researcher concentrates on a sample of people at various stages of the time period he wishes to study in the hope that his sample of people will not be fundamentally different from the other members of the total group. Therefore, instead of following a group of student nurses throughout their training, he will study the group in their first year, he will then focus his attention on a second-year student group and a third-year group. They will not be the same people, but they will all be student nurses. From a research methodological point of view this design has advantages and disadvantages. The advantages are the saving of time and the fact that the members of the particular group studied do not begin to behave differently just because they are being observed and followed through over a period of time. The main disadvantage is generated by the fact that the groups studied comprise different people and the changes observed may be due to those differences rather than to the common experience, such as nurse training, through which they are passing.

Experimental research   The main difference between descriptive and experimental research is that while in the former an existing situation is described, in the latter it is manipulated. As alluded to at the beginning of this chapter, experimental research is necessary if the research findings are to demonstrate a relationship between cause and effect, that is, to predict or explain. Most experimental research designs are based on the principle of an experimental and a control group. The groups are as similar as possible in all respects except that the experimental group receives the input of the factor whose effect is to be studied. This factor is referred to as the 'independent variable'. The groups are then observed with regard to specific predetermined factors called 'dependent variables'. Differences in the dependent variables between the groups can be attributed to the experimental factor. This explanation of experimental research design is deliberately grossly over-simplified. The design of experimental research, of which there are several varieties, is a complex task which demands considerable skill and statistical knowledge.

   The authors consider that readers who wish to understand fully the various methods of setting up an experimental study must study research methodology in greater depth than this book provides, and suggestions for suitable texts are provided at the end of this chapter. An example of a study using an experimental design is that by Paykel and Griffith (1983) who compared the effectiveness for neurotic patients of follow-up care given by community psychiatric nurses with that from traditional psychiatric out-patient attendance.

Probably because of the difficulties and complexities surrounding experimental research, relatively few studies have been undertaken by British nurses. The main difficulty which daunts the potential experimental researcher is that of selecting and keeping constant two similar groups to be studied. The term used by researchers is 'holding variables constant'. The reader will easily recognise the problem of, for example, preserving two groups of patients from all extraneous influences other than that to be studied. For this reason much of the experimental research undertaken by nurses may be more appropriately described as quasi-experimental (Cook & Campbell 1979). Nurse researchers who have attempted such work have been fully cognisant of the problems and have made appropriate allowances in their design and their interpretation of the findings.

Action research

In action research the researcher's focus is a local situation in which he wishes either to solve a local problem or to evaluate the effects of specific change involving the people who are part of the situation. The action researcher does not attempt to hold anything constant, but observes in a systematic manner how the people in the system cope with a local problem or how they adjust to an imposed change. Tierney's research (Tierney 1983) combines the pure experimental design with an action approach. The latter lies in the fact that she involved the nurses actually working on the ward in the toilet training programme. Although her main focus of research was the toileting behaviour of the mentally handicapped patients, she also documented the nursing staff's reactions to the innovation and its effect on ward routine. Moreover, she returned to the ward some time after completion of her research in order to discover whether the toilet training programme had been continued.

The scientific design of action research needs to be as careful as that of other types of research, and all the normal principles relating to the research process apply. Action research has the disadvantage of being applicable only to the specific situation which was studied; it allows for no generalisation. The advantage lies in its better chance of implementation if and where appropriate. An example of this approach is the work of Lathlean & Farmish (1984) who followed an action research protocol in their study of the implementation of a ward sister training scheme.

Methods of data collection in empirical research

In most empirical nursing research the subjects being studied are human beings. There are two main methods, which may be combined, by which one can obtain information which relates to human beings, that is, by observing them or by asking them questions. In this section we have restricted ourselves to discussing these methods and the most frequently used techniques, particularly those which have been used in the research described in later chapters. Other methods of data collection have been developed and the interested reader is referred to the suggested general research texts.

Observation   Observation for research purposes demands skill and scientific rigour. It is easy to see what one expects to see or what one would like to see. The observer has to be trained to observe as reliably as possible; a test of such reliability would be a check by another observer, which is rarely possible. The use of video and audio recording equipment ensures greater reliability by allowing several people to observe and replay the situation after the event and this technological facility is being used increasingly (Macleod Clark 1983). The forms used for recording the observations of the research instruments are also most important. Observations may be recorded inaccurately simply because the recording form is unsuitable or inadequate, but such problems should have come to light in a pilot study. Observation is traditionally divided into two main types, participant and non-participant observation.

Participant observation In participant observation the researcher becomes part of the situation which is being studied. Thus, a nurse researcher may be part of the ward team and record observations in the normal course of the work. An example of participant observation is the work of Janes (1984). The major disadvantage of participant observation is the fact the participation by the researcher in an activity which does not normally include that person makes it an atypical situation. Moreover, there may be ethical problems where a researcher pretends to be part of the system. In addition, a participant observer cannot record observations immediately and has to rely on memory.

Non-participant observation   In non-participant observation, the researcher is 'outside' the working team and attempts to take no part whatever in the activities to be observed. This approach has been used most frequently in nursing research up to now. Macleod Clark (1983) used this method of data collection in the general ward setting, Le May and Redfern (1987) in the geriatric ward setting, and Ashworth (1980) in intensive care units. Many other examples of non-participant observation are referred to in later chapters. The major disadvantage of this type of data collection is the effect which the observer might have on the people being observed, and some procedures have been developed to reduce such possible bias. As it is rarely possible to rule out bias completely, it is important to be aware of it and to make allowances for it in the interpretation of the data which have been collected in this way.

Non-participant observation is usually carried out in one of two ways: continuous observation or activity sampling. Again, it is possible to combine both methods. Continuous observation is the method of choice where the sequence of activities is considered important or when the researcher attempts to obtain the whole picture of a specified time period in a setting where the activities may not follow a set repetitive pattern. Beail (1985) used this type of observation. It is important to emphasise, however, that continuous observation is limited by the length of time the researcher can remain vigilant, and this is rarely for longer than 2 hours at a time.

Activity sampling is a method of observation in which activities are recorded at random time intervals. For example, if one wished to know what type of activities all members of the ward staff were performing during their entire shift, the researcher could record at, say, 15-minute intervals what each member of staff was doing at that time. By using appropriate statistical techniques it is then possible to construct a picture of the total shift period. Continuous observation would have been neither possible nor appropriate for this purpose. The pilot study would demonstrate whether the time intervals selected by the researcher are suitable; no general rule for their selection can be made as the work pattern to be observed is the decisive factor. An example of nursing research in which activity sampling was used is that of Hawthorn (1974).

Operational research is another approach which tends to use activity sampling as a data collecting method. The principle of operational research lies in the construction of an abstract model which is intended to resemble the real-life situation. By mathematical techniques the researcher can manipulate the abstract model and observe the effect of such manipulation. Certain strategies, shown in theory to have a desirable effect, can then be tested in reality. Problems related to the movement of people are particularly amenable to an operational research approach. For example, queueing problems in out-patient departments or the scheduling of learners through the various areas of clinical experience have been successfully handled by operational research.

Asking questions   Questions can be asked in a personal interview or on a postal questionnaire. Both methods have been extensively used in nursing research.

Personal interview   As the term implies, a personal interview is a face-to-face encounter between the researcher and the person being interviewed, the respondent. The interviewer uses an interviewing schedule which lists the questions to be asked and makes provision for the recording of the answers. Researchers distinguish between highly structured and semi-structured interviews. In a highly structured interview the respondent gives one of the possible predetermined answers and has no opportunity to enlarge on any point. In a semi-structured interview the respondent will have some opportunity to answer outside the rigid structure of the schedule; he might, for example, be invited to give his own views on a particular point. Occasionally, the interviewer leaves the interview almost totally open, covering predetermined topics but allowing the respondent a free range of conversation.

The choice of interview between the above alternatives depends on the type of information the researcher wishes to elicit and also on the method of analysis. Thus, if the purpose of the interview is to find out what opinions and views the respondent has on a certain matter, one must give him some freedom in answering. However, such free answers are difficult to handle in the analysis. In most research interviews the interviewing schedule makes provision for some rigidly structured and some free-ranging answers.

Personal interviews are time consuming and, therefore, expensive, but the response is usually better than that obtained from a postal questionnaire.

Postal questionnaires The main distinction between the personal interview method and the postal questionnaire is that in the latter the respondent records the answers himself. Questionnaires have to be most carefully designed so that the respondent has no difficulty in understanding the questions and in knowing exactly how to record his answer. Apart from the saving of time and money, postal questionnaires have the advantage of being free from interviewer bias. Their main disadvantages are that people often do not return them and that there is no opportunity to pursue specific points further. The choice is determined by the type of information required and also by the available time and budget. Thus, where potential respondents are widely scattered geographically, personal interviews would be time consuming and costly.

The advantages and disadvantages of personal interview and postal questionnaire must be carefully weighed up against each other. In a personal interview as well as in a postal questionnaire it is possible to use techniques other than straight questions to obtain certain types of information. Some psychological tests can be incorporated in either method of data collection tool. Attitude tests have been developed which require the respondent to record his answer to set questions. Validated scales are then used to calculate the respective attitudes.

Another method of collecting data is the diary or purpose-designed record. The respondents are asked to record certain information in either a completely free diary style or in a structured form. The diary can either ask for a total description of events over a period of time or for an account of certain happenings within that time period.

From one extreme of leaving respondents entirely free to record their diary events, one can structure a diary by listing events and asking the respondents to tick them as appropriate. It is possible to build time sequences into such a document. Again, the choice will be dependent on the type of information sought and the method of analysis to be conducted.

Summary

This chapter represents a grossly over-simplified account of some of the main research designs and methods. At the end of this section a brief glossary of commonly used research terms has been included. It is hoped that the reader will be able to make links between this information and the studies that are described in detail throughout the book.

References

Ashworth P. (1980) *Time to Care*. London: Royal College of Nursing

Beail N. (1985) The nature of interactions between nursing staff and profoundly mentally handicapped children. *Child: Care Health Development*, **11**, 3, 113–129

Cook T.D. & Campbell D.T. (1979) *Quasi-experimental Designs and Analysis Issues for Research*. Chicago: Rand McNally

Davies C. (1980) *Rewriting Nursing History*. Beckenham: Croom Helm

DHSS (1986) *Neighbourhood Nursing. Report of the Community Nursing Review* (Chairman: J. Cumberlege). London: HMSO

Field P.A. & Morse J.C. (1985) *Nursing Research: the application of qualitative approaches*. Beckenham: Croom Helm

Hawthorn P. (1974) *Nurse, I want my Mummy*. London: Royal College of Nursing

Howard J. & Brooking J. (1987) The career patterns of nursing graduates. *International Journal of Nursing Studies*, **24**, 3, 181–190

Inman V. (1975) *Towards a Theory of Nursing Care*. London: Royal College of Nursing

Janes N. (1984) A postscript to nursing. In Bell C. and Roberts H. (Eds) *Social Researching*. London: Routledge and Kegan Paul

Lathlean J. & Farmish S. (1984) *Ward Sister Training Project. Nursing Education Research Unit Report*. London: Kings College, University of London

Le May A. & Redfern S. (1987) A study of non-verbal communication between nurses and elderly patients. In Fielding P. (Ed.) *Research in the Nursing Care of Elderly People*. Chichester: John Wiley & Sons

McFarlane J. (1970) *The Proper Study of the Nurse*. London: Royal College of Nursing

Macleod Clark J. (1983) An analysis of nurse–patient conversations on surgical wards. In Wilson Barnett J. (Ed.) *Nursing Research. Ten Studies in Patient Care*. Chichester: John Wiley & Sons

Maggs C. (1981) Control mechanisms and the new nurses, 1881–1914. *Nursing Times* Occasional Paper, **25**, 97–100

Melia K. (1982) 'Tell it as it is' – qualitative method and nursing research. *Journal of Advanced Nursing*, **7**, 4, 327–336

Paykel E.S. & Griffith J. (1983) *Community Psychiatric Nursing for Neurotic Patients*. London: Royal College of Nursing

Robinson S., Golden J. & Bradley S. (1983) *A Study of the Role and Responsibility of the Midwife. Nursing Education Research Report No. 1*. London: King's College, University of London

RCN (1985) *The Education of Nurses: a new dispensation*. Commission of Nursing Education. London: Royal College of Nursing

Schröck R. (1977) *The Ongoing Process of Re-appraisal. An Investigation into the Principles of Health Visiting*. London: Council for Education and Training of Health Visitors

Smith J. (1981) The idea of health: a philosophical inquiry. *Advances in Nursing Science*, **3**, 43

Tierney A.J. (1983) Toilet training. *Nursing Times*, **69**, 1740–1745

Williams K. (1974) Ideologies of nursing: their meanings and implications. *Nursing Times* Occasional paper, **8**, 8, 74

A selection of general research methods texts

Cahoon M. (Ed.) (1987) *Recent Advances in Nursing – Research Methodology*. Edinburgh: Churchill Livingstone

Cormack D. (1984) *The Research Process in Nursing*. Oxford: Blackwell Scientific Publishers

Fawcett J. & Downs F.S. (1986) *The Relationship of Theory and Research*. Connecticut: Appleton Century Crofts

Field P.A. & Morse J.M. (1985) *Nursing Research. The Application of Qualitative Approaches*. Beckenham: Croom Helm

Leininger M. (Ed) (1985) *Qualitative Research Methods in Nursing*. New York: Grune and Stratton

Munhall P.L. & Oiler C.J. (1986) *Nursing Research—A Qualitative Perspective*. Connecticut: Appleton Century Crofts

Open University (1979) *Research Methods in Education and the Social Sciences. Blocks 1–8*. Milton Keynes: Open University Press.

Polit D. & Hungler B. (1983) *Nursing Research Principles and Methods*, 2nd Edition. Philadelphia: Lippincott Co.
Polit D. & Hungler B. (1985) *Essentials of Nursing Research*, 2nd Edition. Philadelphia: Lippincott Co.
Reid N. & Boore J. (1987) *Research Methods and Statistics in Health Care*, London: Edward Arnold
Seaman C. & Verhonick P. (1982) *Research Methods for Undergraduate Students in Nursing*, 2nd Edition. New York: Appleton Century Crofts
Shelley S.I. (1984) *Research Methods in Nursing and Health*. Boston: Little, Brown & Co.
Treece E.W. & Treece J.W. Jr. (1982) *Elements of Research in Nursing*, St Louis: C.V. Mosby

Glossary of research terms

Bias	Distortion of the findings resulting from an undesirable influence.
Cohort	An identified group of subjects who are being studied over a period of time.
Data	Facts or phenomena recorded specifically in the course of the research process.
Demographic data	Information about the characteristics of human populations.
Hypothesis	Statement of a relationship which is suggested by knowledge or observation but has not yet been proved or disproved.
Interview:	
structured	An interview which is conducted by means of set questions with a predetermined range of possible responses.
semi-structured	An interview which is conducted by means of set questions but which allows for some flexibility either in the question or in the range of responses.
unstructured	An interview which allows for spontaneous questions and/or free responses.
Mean value/score	The average value or score.
Null hypothesis	Statement which predicts that there will be no significant differences between observations.
Pilot study	Preliminary study intended to test the proposed method for a main study.
Probability	Used in relation to chance occurrences. A research finding which is indicated as having a 'probability' of less than 0.01 ($p<0.01$) means

that the finding was likely to have occurred by mere chance in fewer than 1 in 100 instances.

Random sample
Result of a systematic selection of units from a population where each unit has an equal chance of being selected. A unit can be an individual, a hospital, a medical record, etc.

Research tool/ instrument
Purpose-designed medium, such as questionnaire, used for the collection of research data.

Response rate
Percentage of those approached who actually participated in the study.

Sampling
Method of selecting a certain number of units from a total population.

Statistical significance
Relating to a finding shown by appropriate statistical tests to be unlikely to be due purely to chance.

Theory
A specific set of propositions, developed in any scientific discipline, which is used to explain certain phenomena or events.

Variable
Any factor, characteristic or attribute under study which may distinguish the units within a population from each other, such as qualifications of nurses or diagnoses of patients.

We hope that readers will draw our attention to other terms which could be included in the glossary in future editions.

Part II: Research into the Care of Specific Groups of Patients and Clients

Introduction

Jill Macleod Clark and Lisbeth Hockey

This section of the book contains six chapters, each of which gives a descriptive overview of some of the research which has been undertaken in a particular area of nursing. These chapters are not intended to present a comprehensive or definitive review of the research in each area, nor do they claim to cover every patient or client group. This would not be possible in a book like this. Instead the author of each chapter has attempted to give readers a taste of the research which has been carried out, to illuminate some of the critical issues related to the care of each group of patients or clients, and to identify those areas which require further research.

The over-riding purpose of this book is to stimulate nurses to think critically about nursing and to become increasingly research minded. The emphasis therefore is on helping readers to become aware of the research that exists and to utilise research findings in practice, where relevant. However, we hope that readers may become more conversant with the research process and research methods as a result of reading this book. For this reason, one or two research studies are presented in some detail in each chapter, structured under the headings of Main research question(s); Research design and method; Main findings; and Implications.

Main research question(s) All research should start from a research problem or research question(s). The main research question(s) have been singled out for each piece of research, which has been presented in summary form.

Research design and method The design of any research

project will depend on the type of question being asked. The method used will to some extent determine the level of answers the researcher will find to the research questions asked. As indicated in Chapter 2, where an overview of research methods and design can be found, some designs and approaches are intended to describe a situation, others to explain and some to predict. In each type of design the researcher can choose from a variety of methods to collect the required information or data.

Main findings   When the items of information or data have been collected, they are structured or ordered in a systematic way and then analysed in order to produce results or findings.

Implications   The purpose of all research is to generate new knowledge and understanding. The implications of the findings from any piece of research are what can be learnt from the study. In the following chapters, authors have suggested some of the implications which arise from each of the studies they have described. Again, the implications of research are never definitive. There may be many alternative ways of looking at the material and the findings can be interpreted from different perspectives, although it is essential to go back and read the original research report in order to make such judgements.

The material in this section of the book covers the care of a wide variety of groups of patients and clients. The research that has been included inevitably represents only a small proportion of that available. It is hoped that readers will be inspired to find out more about research in their particular fields of interest by following up the references and reading some of the original reports.

Chapter 3

The Care of Elderly People

PAULINE FIELDING

The nursing care of elderly people as a specialty in its own right is still in its infancy, but judging from the growth in the research literature over the last 25 years, we can conclude that it is growing up quickly. This chapter will review some of that literature but will be necessarily selective in order to give the reader an overview of the range of issues that are encompassed. Omission of any particular topic does not indicate a lack of research literature or a judgement of unimportance. A recent collection of British geriatric nursing research studies can be seen in Fielding (1987).

Researchers have recognised the importance in recent years of attempting to measure the outcomes of nursing care. With elderly patients, outcome in terms of quality of life is sometimes more important than quantitative improvement in physical status. We should recognise, however, that there is not a very clear line dividing the two aspects. Some researchers have focused on patient satisfaction (Raphael 1977, 1979; Forgan Morle 1984), other on sources of stress (Davies & Peters 1983). All, however, look to improved communication as a means of preventing potential distress or dissatisfaction.

The measurement of outcome in relation to a specific treatment or type of care environment has taken a new turn. There is now a move away from considering the patient's pathological disease process, towards measuring what the patient can do in functional terms. Many researchers have used some kind of activities of daily living (ADL) scale in order to assess treatment outcome in the care of elderly people (Applegate *et al.* 1983; Lefton *et al.* 1983; Jackson 1984; Stewart 1980; Fielding 1987). Jackson, for example, used Plutchik's Geriatric Rating Scale and Katz's Index of ADL to show the effect of a rehabilitation pilot project for elderly patients on an acute medical unit. Interestingly, there were significant changes in behaviour for the patients involved. This is one of the few studies which addresses the issue of specialised versus general wards for old people and is an example of an area which merits further detailed investigation.

In modern geriatric nursing practice a great deal of emphasis is placed on maintaining the elderly person's independence for as long as possible. The ability to remain independent can be affected by psychological or physiological factors. The psychological impact of illness and hospitalisation has been reviewed by Wilson-Barnett (1979) and Davies and Peters (1983), who have considered nurses' and elderly patients' perceptions of what are considered to be stressful situations. Davies and Peters interviewed 25 elderly patients and their nurses using a 16-item stress scale which covered such areas as noise, doctors, visitors, toiletting, privacy, loneliness, nursing care and medicines. Patients were generally complimentary about the care they received and there was overall agreement between nurses and patients as to what patients found stressful. However, whereas nurses considered that the stress of some of these situations (noise on the ward, doctors' visits, and toiletting) decreased over time, patients rated the stressfulness at the same level or even higher as time went on. This suggests that nurses may not always be in tune with their patients and may underestimate the effect of prolonged hospitalisation. Davies and Peters conclude their report by suggesting that the introduction of a problem-orientated approach to nursing care should increase the congruence of nurses' and patients' perceptions.

The proportion of elderly people in the population is increasing steadily and this demographic trend is likely to continue in the foreseeable future. The number of dependent elderly people is also likely to increase unless strenuous attempts are made actively to encourage rehabilitation and independence. It is estimated that approximately two-thirds of old people in geriatric wards are incontinent, three-quarters need help with mobility, more than two-thirds need help with washing and dressing, and approximately one-fifth are spoonfed (Miller 1985). The speculation that much of the dependency found amongst geriatric patients could be caused by outdated and inappropriate nursing practice led to a research study by Miller (1985) which is described below.

TITLE OF ARTICLE: A Study of the Dependency of Elderly Patients in Wards using different Methods of Nursing Care

Main research question   To what extent is dependency in elderly patients influenced by the methods of organising nursing care?

Research design and method   Miller compared two wards in each of three hospitals where the patients were similar in terms of dependency. The wards were similar in size, in admission policy, type of patient, staffing levels and training/non-training areas, but differed in terms of the methods used to organise care. In all, 168 patients were studied, of ages ranging from 61 to 97 years (average 80 years). The instrument used to measure the degree of dependency was the CAPE – Clifton Assessment Procedures for the Elderly (Pattie & Gilleard 1979). This is a behaviour rating scale which, when completed, indicates the degree of impairment and dependency of the person with regard to their physical needs, apathy, social disturbance, communication difficulties and incontinence. Scores achieved by patients in each of the wards were compared. In addition, one ward was studied over a period of 2 years. At the start of the project the care was organised by means of task allocation, but over the next 2 years a programme of individualised nursing care was introduced.

Dependency levels of the patients were compared before and after the new programme was introduced.

Main findings   At the start of the study it was found that the method of nursing care did not affect the behaviour ratings of patients who had been in hospital less than a month. However, long-stay patients who had been in hospital for more than 1 month were significantly more dependent if they were nursed by task allocation rather than by the individualised nursing process method. More evidence came from the study over 2 years of the one ward where the method of care was changed. When the nursing care on this ward was organised by means of task allocation, the dependency score of the 27 long-stay patients was high. Over the next 2 years, after a programme of individualised nursing care had been introduced, the dependency of the patients decreased to a level comparable with other individualised care wards. Miller claims that as there were no other major changes of policy or staffing levels, the increased independence of the patients was the result of the change in nursing practice.

Implications   This study showed not only that outdated nursing practices increased the dependency of patients, but also that they were associated with an increased mortality and less likelihood of discharge. Patients in the traditional wards stayed longer, their chances of dying were marginally greater, and they were less likely to be discharged than those patients in individualised care wards. Miller also used the findings of her study to question the adequacy of nurse staffing formulae which assume that nursing care arises as a direct result of the patient's illness and dependency. Her research certainly underlines the need for every patient to be given an individual plan of care.

It is also clear that more attention should be given to the outcomes of organising care in more innovative and less stereotyped ways. The potential long-term benefits of such approaches in terms of increasing the independence of elderly patients cannot be overestimated.

Another central issue in the care of elderly patients is that of communication. Many such patients are lonely and isolated and a high proportion have sensory deficits which render communication more difficult (Macleod Clark 1986). There have been a number of studies of verbal communication between nurses and patients and most of these have concentrated on the frequency and duration of the interactions. In general it has been found that the communication is limited in quantity and quality. Wells (1980) demonstrated that the majority of conversations between nurses and elderly patients were perfunctory and tended to be related to tasks or procedures.

Most educational programmes on caring for old people emphasise the importance of nurses holding appropriate attitudes because it is generally felt that attitudes determine behaviour and influence the nursing care and ultimate well-being of patients. Fielding (1986) has reviewed this literature in depth and, in a study of student nurses' attitudes towards old people in hospital, concluded that whilst emphasis was placed on talking to patients, the nurses had few skills to bring to this activity. In consequence the positive attitudes they held towards elderly patients were not borne out by the nurses' communication. Luker (1981) also highlights the importance of attitudes and argues that health visitors lack an appropriate frame of reference for caring for the elderly. This is an area which merits further investigation given the increasing numbers of ageing people living in the community.

A further aspect of communication and attitudes to which nurses need to pay more attention in the future is that of ethnicity. As ethnic groups become more established in our communities, more of their old people will be cared for in hospital wards, and as yet research data on communication patterns between such groups and health service personnel are few. In a Canadian study, Jones and Van Amelsvoort Jones (1986) examined verbal communication patterns between immigrants, Canadian-born and Anglo-born elderly people in a longterm care home. There were some disturbing patterns of interaction noted in this study. It should perhaps be noted that during the 72 hours of the study, only 850 words were spoken to the 36 residents in total and commands were the most frequent form of speech. This is clearly an area where further research is merited.

Non-verbal communication is also very important in the care of elderly people and research in this field has increased in recent years. Much of this work is American, but a recent British study by Le May and Redfern (1987), which examined non-verbal communication between nurses and elderly patients, suggests that most nurse–patient touching was instrumental or task related in nature as opposed to being expressive. Further research is therefore needed in the area of non-verbal communication to assess the potential benefits of incorporating increased contact and touch in the care of elderly people.

A specialised use of communication skills is in the field of reality orientation. This encompasses a range of communication techniques which confirm and re-affirm the person's sense of identity in a particular place and time. Early work (Holden & Woods 1982; Merchant & Saxby 1981) suggested that improvements in cognitive performance could result from reality orientation programmes with patients in a long-stay geriatric ward. After 4 months they found that patients scoring in the medium range of the Holden Communication Scale showed most improvement. There was little change for both high and low scorers, suggesting that severity of cognitive impairment at the outset was a reliable predictor of likely change in response to a reality orientation programme.

These findings clearly have implications for nurses caring for elderly people. In particular, attention should be focused on the need to improve methods of the nursing assessment of patients' cognitive abilities.

Summary

Currently old people occupy more than half of all hospital beds in the UK. As numbers of elderly people in the population increase, the need for nurses to develop a research-based approach to the care of these patients will also grow. One important area for future research is the exploration of the most appropriate setting for the care of elderly patients. For example, it is not clear whether care is best undertaken in designated geriatric wards or in mixed wards. Further studies are needed on methods of encouraging independence in elderly people, in particular, effective strategies for enabling old people to remain in the community. Ross (1988) has investigated aspects of medication and information sharing between health professionals and elderly people in the community, and Dawson (1987) has described a night sitting service for those old people with senile dementia. Other areas which would merit further study include an examination of effective approaches to rehabilitation and increasing self-care, diet and nutrition in relation to elderly patients. The opportunities for research are limitless.

References

Applegate W.B., Akins D., Vanderzwaag R., Thoni K. & Baker M.G. (1983) A geriatric rehabilitation and assessment unit in a community hospital. *Journal of the American Geriatric Society*, **31**, 4, 206–210

Davies A.D.M. & Peters M. (1983) Stresses of hospitalisation in the elderly; nurses and patients perceptions. *Journal of Advanced Nursing*, **8**, 99–105

Dawson J. (1987) Evaluation of a community-based night sitter service. In Fielding P. (Ed.) *Research in the Nursing Care of Elderly People*. Chichester: John Wiley & Sons

Fielding P. (1986) *Attitudes Revisited*. London: Royal College of Nursing

Fielding P. (1987) *Research in the Nursing Care of Elderly People.* Chichester: John Wiley & Sons

Forgan Morle K.M. (1984) Patient satisfaction: care of the elderly. *Journal of Advanced Nursing*, **9**, 71–76

Holden U.P. & Woods R. (1982) *Reality Orientation: Psychological Approaches to the Confused Elderly.* London: Churchill Livingstone

Jackson M.F. (1984) Geriatric rehabilitation on an acute-care medical unit. *Journal of Advanced Nursing*, **9**, 441–448

Jones D.C. & Van Amelsvoort Jones G.M.M. (1986) Communication patterns between nursing staff and the ethnic elderly in a long-term care facility. *Journal of Advanced Nursing*, **11**, 265–272

Le May A.C. & Redfern S.J. (1987) A study of non-verbal communication between nurses and elderly patients. In Fielding P. (Ed.) *Research in the Nursing Care of Elderly People.* Chichester: John Wiley & Sons

Lefton E., Bonstelle S. & Frengley J.D. (1983) Success with an in-patient geriatric unit; a controlled study of outcome and follow-up. *Journal of the American Geriatric Society*, **31**, 3, 149–155

Luker K. (1981) The role of the health visitor. In Kinniard J. *et al.* Edinburgh: Churchill Livingstone

Macleod Clark J. (1986) In Redfern S.J. (Ed.) *Nursing Elderly People.* Edinburgh: Churchill Livingstone.

Merchant M. & Saxby P. (1981) Reality orientation; a way forward. *Nursing Times*, **77**, 33

Miller A. (1985) A study of the dependency of elderly patients in wards using different methods of nursing care. *Age and Ageing*, **14**, 132–138

Pattie A.H. & Gilleard C.J. (1979) *CAPE scales. Manual of the Clifton Assessment Procedures for the Elderly.* Essex: Hodder and Stoughton

Raphael W. (1977) *Patients and their Hospitals.* London: King Edward's Fund for London

Raphael W. (1979) *Old People in Hospital.* London: King Edward's Fund

Ross F.M. (1988) Information sharing between patients, nurses and doctors. In Johnson R. (Ed.) *Excellence in Nursing.* Recent Advances Series. Edinburgh: Churchill Livingstone

Stewart C.P.U. (1980) A prediction score for geriatric rehabilitation prospects. *Rheumatology and Rehabilitation*, **19**, 239–245.

Wells T.J. (1980) *Problems in Geriatric Nursing Care.* Edinburgh: Churchill Livingstone

Wilson-Barnett J. (1979) *Stress in Hospital: Patients' Psychological Reactions to Illness and Health Care.* Edinburgh: Churchill Livingstone

Chapter 4

The Care of Psychiatric Patients

JULIA I. BROOKING

This chapter gives a brief overview of research concerning psychiatric nursing. Inevitably, a short chapter can do no more than point out some important studies, and much interesting work has had to be omitted. Most of the studies cited are British. There are major differences between psychiatric nursing practice in Britain and abroad (Reed, in press) and foreign literature may not be be readily available. Research by psychiatric nurses into psychiatric nursing is of relatively recent origin, but psychiatric nurses have long drawn on research carried out by workers in other disciplines, particularly work derived from psychology, sociology, psychiatry and the neurosciences. Role overlap among members of multidisciplinary teams is common in psychiatry and therefore much research concerning the nature of mental disorders and methods of therapy is relevant to nursing. Examples include studies on the effects of 'expressed emotion' in precipitating schizophrenic relapse (Vaughn & Leff 1976) and work evaluating various types of psychotherapy, reviewed by Garfield and Bergin (1986).

Recent British psychiatric nursing studies are wide ranging and have been reviewed in Brooking (1986). For clarity, the main areas of study can be divided into seven categories.

1. Role of the nurse

Towell (1975) used participant observation to examine nursing practice in admission and psychogeriatric wards and a therapeutic community. The nurses' role varied in each of the settings, and nurses' treatment ideology was largely determined

39

by doctors' therapeutic orientation. Cormack (1976) carried out a descriptive study of the work of charge nurses in acute admission wards and found a large gulf between actual and prescribed roles. He found no evidence of nurses taking an active therapeutic role. In his more recent research, Cormack (1983) adopted an evaluative approach when describing the role of the ward-based psychiatric nurse. Using the Critical Incident Technique (Flanagan 1954), he collected thousands of examples of effective and ineffective nursing actions from patients, nurses and doctors. These were used to develop a framework within which the nursing role could be classified. He found the role to be multidimensional including therapeutic, administrative, technical, educational and other components. Cormack's (1983) classification has important implications for nursing education and for evaluating care.

2. Community psychiatric nursing

This is an area of practice which has attracted considerable research interest. Descriptive analyses include the work of Parnell (1978) and Sladden (1979). Skidmore (1986) examined the relationship between community psychiatric nurses' (CPN) base-locations and methods of practice. He studied hospital and primary health care-based CPN teams, but found no differences in intervention styles. White (1986) studied relationships between CPNs and general practitioners (GPs) and found great diversity. Not surprisingly, relationships with and referrals to CPNs seemed to be at least partly a function of the relationships negotiated between the individuals concerned. One large study led by a Professor of Psychiatry (Paykel & Griffith 1983) evaluated the work of CPNs by comparing outcomes for their patients with those attending a conventional out-patient service. This is described in detail below.

TITLE OF BOOK: *Community Psychiatric Nursing for Neurotic Patients*

Main research question   What is the efficacy of follow-up care of neurotic patients by CPNs as opposed to traditional psychiatric out-patient follow-up, in terms of symptoms, social adjustment, family burden, consumer satisfaction and costs?

Research design and methods   The design of the study was a prospective, randomised, controlled trial. Subjects were predominantly middle-aged women suffering from depression and anxiety, who had been out-patient attenders for at least 6 months, or were about to be discharged from in-patient or day-patient care and who required continuing care. Patients were randomly assigned either to CPN care or out-patient care. Ninety-nine patients entered the study and 71 completed 18 months of follow-up assessments. Research assessments were carried out on entry to the study and at 6-monthly intervals to 18 months. These included data on symptoms, performance of social and economic roles, services received, patient satisfaction and family burden.

Main findings   There were no significant differences between the two groups with regard to symptoms, social role performance and degree of family burden. Satisfaction with treatment was significantly higher in the CPN group. Nurses were rated as significantly more easy to talk to, interested, pleasant, caring and relaxing than psychiatrists. This effect increased over time. CPNs achieved a greater number of discharges than routine out-patient care and economic analysis showed that over the whole study period CPN care was less expensive.

Implications   These findings support the continuing development of CPN services, as care by CPNs produced as good clinical benefits as out-patient attendance. The researchers were concerned to point out that the CPNs worked as part of multidisciplinary teams and received clinical support from psychiatrists when necessary, and the study was not therefore a comparison of the efficacy of two professional groups. Patient satisfaction was higher in the CPN group and patients expressed particular satisfaction with the home location, information given by the nurse and the nurse–patient relationship. Although important, consumer satisfaction is a limited goal in itself, unless clinical efficacy can also be demonstrated. Although case studies were produced to illustrate the process of care, the main emphasis of the study was on the measurement of patient outcomes. It is clearly equally important to identify the structures within which care takes place and the processes of care, in order that relationships between structure, process and outcome can be elicited. Methodologically this study is important in demonstrating the applicability of controlled evaluative studies to nursing practice research.

3. Behaviour therapy nursing

A number of studies led by Professor Isaac Marks have evaluated the work of nurse therapists. Marks *et al.* (1975, 1978) found that clinical outcomes for their patients compared well with those obtained by psychiatrists, psychologists and medical students. Marks *et al.* (1977) found that the nurse therapists' competence to assess, diagnose and plan treatment matched that of psychiatrists. A large study to evaluate the efficacy of nurse therapists in primary care was reported by Marks (1985). Sixty-six patients who were considered suitable for behaviour therapy were randomly assigned either to nurse behaviour therapy or care by their own GPs, who had no specific training in behavioural techniques. Patients treated by nurse therapy were significantly superior to the GP group on various clinical measures up to 2 years follow-up. Patients treated by GPs did not make useful gains until transferred to nurse therapist treatment. A cost–benefit analysis (Ginsberg *et al.* 1985) showed that it cost less to treat suitable neurotic disorders by nurse therapy than to leave them untreated. Marks (1985) found that nurse therapists were well accepted by GPs and their opinions were sought on general psychiatric matters. A national follow-up survey of the career patterns of qualified nurse therapists was carried out by Brooker and Brown (1986). In summary, they found that nurse therapists organise and locate their work in a variety of ways. They value their independence and find the work satisfying, but are frustrated at being unable to advance their careers.

4. Nurse–patient communication

Research in this area includes the work of Altschul (1972) who observed contacts between patients and nurses. She could not obtain any picture of treatment ideologies prevailing amongst nurses, who insisted that interactions were just common sense. Patients valued the availability of nurses and experienced relationships as helpful. MacIlwaine (1983) studied the communication patterns of female neurotic patients with nurses in psychiatric units of general hospitals. Interactions tended to be very brief and mainly concerned practical and administrative matters. There was no planned therapeutic interaction and talking to patients was seen as a low priority activity. Street (1982) found similar results in a smaller scale study.

5. Nursing education

Various aspects of psychiatric nursing education have been studied. Brooking (1985) examined provision for advanced education and concluded that there was a shortage of high-level educational opportunities for psychiatric nurses. Muir-Cochrane (1986) surveyed the psychiatric nursing component of degree/RGN courses. Gournay (1986) measured changes in nurses' attitudes after undertaking post-basic courses. He found that trainee nurse therapists were less conservative and favoured a more psychological, less organic approach to treatment than psychiatric nurses generally. In interviews with 21 RMN students, Powell (1982) revealed that students thought the ability to relate to patients was important, but could not be taught, and used existing skills improved through ward experience. Their teaching emphasised the dangers of over-involvement and manipulation by patients. Research on student nurse socialisation was carried out by Davis (1986) using the repertory grid technique (Kelly 1955). He provided valuable insights into students' perceptions of themselves and of psychiatric nursing and made recommendations for helping students to cope with the stressful process of becoming psychiatric nurses.

6. Care of the elderly mentally infirm

Several researchers have used the case study approach to examine the quality of care given to elderly mentally infirm people in psychogeriatric wards. Examples include the work of Towell (1975), Savage et al. (1979), Unwin (1981) and Miller (1978). All these studies found that staff contact with patients related mainly to physical care and there was little social interaction or attempts to meet patients' emotional needs. These researchers found that patients were inactive and under-stimulated and there were few attempts to individualise care.

7. Nursing interventions for specific patient problems

Although crucial for practice, there have been few studies concerning the effectiveness of particular nursing interventions. Towell and Harries (1979) described a series of small-scale developments and evaluations in a psychiatric hospital and demonstrated that innovation can originate from clinical nurses. Gordon (1986), in a British replication of her American research, evaluated a group intervention for depressed women facilitated by psychiatric nurses. Women who attended the series of group meetings showed a significant decrease in depression and increase in self-esteem compared with women who did not attend the group. This demonstrates the ability of nurses to lead a successful treatment programme. Research reported by Brooking and Minghella (1987) explored the effectiveness of psychiatric nurses in assessing and caring for patients following parasuicide and compared the service provided by nurses with more traditional methods of treatment. This illustrates how a service innovation may be established on a pilot basis and systematically evaluated.

Discussion

Psychiatric nursing research is still at an early stage of development and many studies are small scale and methodologically and conceptually simple. Many of the studies in this chapter describe inadequate practices, but research developing and evaluating new practices is rare. This reflects both psychiatric nurses' lack of educational preparation to carry out major studies (Brooking 1985) and difficulties in obtaining funding. Researchers have been attracted to work on specialist subjects which still involve a minority of nurses and patients, such as nurse behaviour therapy and community psychiatric nursing. Basic questions about the effectiveness of practices in institutional settings remain to be answered and most nursing is still planned at an intuitive rather than a scientific level. The care of acutely psychotic and institutionalised patients is particularly under-researched, with rare exceptions such as MacDonald (1985), who interviewed nurses working in rehabilitation and long-stay wards to identify their perceptions of patients' needs and problems. Methodological work is particularly needed to provide the tools of research as few objective methods of patient assessment and evaluation exist. Methods of measuring the structure and process of care, as well as patient outcomes, also need to be developed. There has been little attempt to identify priorities for future psychiatric nursing research. In an American study, Ventura and Woligora-Serafin (1981) demonstrated the feasibility of the Delphi technique (see Lindeman 1975) in identifying psychiatric nursing research needs. They found that the highest rated items were: factors contributing to repeated hospital admissions; the role of the nurse after discharge from hospital; patient compliance; and factors related to staff burnout. The extent to which these findings would reflect British psychiatric nurses' priorities for research is not yet known.

References

Altschul A. (1972) *Patient–Nurse Interaction: A Study of Interaction Patterns in Acute Psychiatric Wards.* Edinburgh: Churchill Livingstone

Brooker C. & Brown M. (1986) National follow-up survey of practising nurse therapists. In Brooking J.I. (Ed.) *Psychiatric Nursing Research.* Chichester: John Wiley & Sons

Brooking J.I. (1985) Advanced psychiatric nursing education in Britain. *Journal of Advanced Nursing*, **10**, 455–468

Brooking J.I. (Ed.) (1986) *Psychiatric Nursing Research.* Chichester: John Wiley & Sons

Brooking J.I. & Minghella E. (1987) Parasuicide. *Nursing Times*, **83**, 21, 40–43

Cormack D.F. (1976) *Psychiatric Nursing Observed.* London: Royal College of Nursing

Cormack D.F. (1983) *Psychiatric Nursing Described.* Edinburgh: Churchill Livingstone

Davis B.D. (1986) The strain of training: being a student psychiatric nurse. In Brooking J.I. (Ed.) *Psychiatric Nursing Research.* Chichester: John Wiley & Sons

Flanagan J.C. (1954) The critical incident technique. *Psychological Bulletin*, **51**, 4, 327–358

Garfield S.L. & Bergin A.E. (Eds) (1986) *Handbook of Psychotherapy and Behaviour Change*, 3rd Edn. New York: John Wiley & Sons

Ginsberg G., Marks I. & Waters H. (1985) A controlled cost–benefit analysis. In Marks I. (Ed.) *Psychiatric Nurse Therapists in Primary Care.* London: Royal College of Nursing

Gordon V. (1986) Reducing depression in women: research in the USA and GB. In Brooking J.I. (Ed.) *Psychiatric Nursing Research.* Chichester: John Wiley & Sons

Gournay K. (1986) A pilot study of nurses' attitudes with relation to post-basic training. In Brooking J.I. (Ed.) *Psychiatric Nursing Research.* Chichester: John Wiley & Sons

Kelly G.A. (1955) *The Psychology of Personal Constructs,* Vols. 1 and 2. New York: Norton

Lindeman C. (1975) Delphi survey of priorities in clinical nursing research. *Nursing Research,* **24,** 434–441

MacDonald H. (1985) *A Humane and Dignified Task? An Exploratory Study of Nursing in Psychiatric Rehabilitation.* Project submitted for BSc (Hons) Nursing Studies, Chelsea College (copies in the University of London libraries at King's College and St George's Medical School)

MacIlwaine H. (1983) The communication patterns of female neurotic patients with nursing staff in psychiatric units of general hospitals. In Wilson-Barnett J. (Ed.) *Nursing Research: Ten Studies in Patient Care.* Chichester: John Wiley & Sons

Marks I.M. (1985) *Psychiatric Nurse Therapists in Primary Care.* London: Royal College of Nursing

Marks I.M., Bird J. & Lindley P. (1978) Psychiatric nurse therapists 1978 – developments and implications. *Behavioural Psychotherapy,* **6,** 25–35

Marks I.M., Connolly J., Hallam R. & Philpott R. (1975) Nurse therapists in behavioural psychotherapy. *British Medical Journal,* **iii,** 144–148

Marks I.M., Connolly J., Hallam R. & Philpott R. (1977) *Nursing in Behavioural Psychotherapy: An Advanced Clinical Role for Nurses.* London: Royal College of Nursing

Miller A.E. (1978) *Evaluation of the Care Provided for Patients with Dementia in Six Hospital Wards.* Unpublished MSc thesis, University of Manchester

Muir-Cochrane E. (1986) An examination of the psychiatric nursing component of degree/RGN courses in Britain. In Brooking J.I. (Ed.) *Psychiatric Nursing Research.* Chichester: John Wiley & Sons

Parnell J.W. (1978) *Community Psychiatric Nursing: a Descriptive Study.* London: Queen's Nursing Institute

Paykel E.S. & Griffith J.H. (1983) *Community Psychiatric Nursing for Neurotic Patients.* London: Royal College of Nursing

Powell D. (1982) *Learning to Relate: A Study of Student Psychiatric Nurses' Views of their Preparation and Training.* London: Royal College of Nursing

Reed M.A. (In press) Global perspective. In Brooking J.I. (Ed.) *Textbook of Psychiatric Nursing.* Edinburgh: Churchill Livingstone

Savage B., Widdowson T. & Wright T. (1979) Improving the care of the elderly. In Towell D. & Harries C. (Eds) *Innovation in Patient Care*. London: Croom Helm

Skidmore D. (1986) The effectiveness of community psychiatric nursing teams and base-locations. In Brooking J.I. (Ed.) *Psychiatric Nursing Research*. Chichester: John Wiley & Sons

Sladden S. (1979) *Psychiatric Nursing in the Community: A Study of the Working Situation*. Edinburgh: Churchill Livingstone

Street C.G. (1982) *An Investigation of the Priority on Nurse–Patient Interaction by Psychiatric Nurses*. Project submitted for BSc (Hons) Nursing Studies, Chelsea College (copies in the University of London libraries at King's College and St George's Medical School)

Towell D. (1975) *Understanding Psychiatric Nursing: A Sociological Study of Modern Psychiatric Nursing Practice*. London: Royal College of Nursing

Towell D. & Harries C. (1979) *Innovation in Patient Care*. London: Croom Helm

Unwin K. (1981) *A Case Study to Investigate Problems Faced by Nurses on a Psychogeriatric Ward*. Project submitted for BSc (Hons) Nursing Studies, Chelsea College (copies in the University of London libraries at King's College and St George's Medical School)

Vaughn C.E. & Leff J.P. (1976) The influence of family and social factors on the course of psychiatric illness: a comparison of schizophrenic and depressed neurotic patients. *British Journal of Psychiatry*, **129**, 125–137

Ventura M.R. & Woligora-Serafin B. (1981) Study priorities identified by nurses in mental health settings. *International Journal of Nursing Studies*, **18**, 41–46

White E. (1986) Factors influencing general practitioners to refer patients to community psychiatric nurses. In Brooking J.I. (ed.). *Psychiatric Nursing Research*. Chichester: John Wiley & Sons

Chapter 5

The Care of People with a Mental Handicap

Philip Darbyshire

Although the amount of research carried out by nurses has been increasing steadily since the early 1970s, comparatively few such research studies have been undertaken in the field of mental handicap. The vast majority of research in mental handicap over the last 20 years has been concerned with behavioural management programmes based upon behaviour therapy principles.

These studies have without doubt made a valuable contribution to the care of the mentally handicapped. Examples of such research include Paton and Petrusev's (1974) attempt to increase the verbal communication patterns of moderately handicapped adolescents by implementing a structured teaching programme. Similarly, in a study by Tierney (1973), an experiment was designed using behaviour modification techniques to toilet train a group of severely handicapped residents in their usual ward environment. She found that there was a significant reduction of incontinence achieved by the experimental group, with a consequent decrease in the amount of linen required and in the amount of nurses' time being devoted to the management of incontinence and toileting. Improvements were also noted in the general level of functioning of those in the experimental group which might suggest that nurses' efforts directed at one area of care may generalise to produce improvements in other areas.

In such a brief overview of recent research it has been necessary to be selective and the studies highlighted in this chapter cover the two vital areas of nurse–resident interaction and community care.

Interactions between nurses and mentally handicapped residents

In a memorable passage, Blackwell (1979) claims that:

> Neither the size of a residential facility, nor its budget, nor the qualification of its staff, nor its programme objectives determine the institution's success in promoting health or human development. While these factors influence the likelihood of a healthy environment, the most significant factor is the quality of human contact received by residents.

Nurse–resident interaction is a crucial issue which underpins all other aspects of working with mentally handicapped people. Poor quality or inadequate interaction will cause important opportunities for social contact and learning to be lost. At a more basic level, the lack of good quality interaction can condemn a profoundly multiply handicapped person to a life almost devoid of any human contact.

Oswin (1978) drew attention to the paucity of stimuli and attention given to profoundly handicapped children who were living in long-stay hospitals. She found that they received an average 1 hour of physical care and 5 minutes of 'mothering' attention in a 10-hour period. More recent studies have found similar patterns of interaction. Cullen *et al.* (1983) studied interactions between staff and 10 residents within a medium-sized (approximately 120 residents) mental handicap institution. They found that each resident was likely to have some reaction to his behaviour on average once every 25 minutes, and that the interaction with a carer that resulted was likely to last for less than 10 seconds. The researchers felt that as the level of interactions between staff and residents was so low, it was difficult to draw conclusions from the study. A similar study of 48 mental handicap residents by Allan and Goodbody (1984) found that on average residents had contact with nursing staff for only 20 minutes out of a possible 12½ hours and received no attention for 93% of the time.

Felce *et al.* (1985) compared interaction patterns between residents living in small community houses and in large mental handicap hospitals. They demonstrated that a group of severely and profoundly mentally handicapped adults who were living in small community houses spent a greater proportion of their time in interaction than did those who lived in institutions.

Beail (1985) has undertaken an in-depth study of interaction between nursing staff and mentally handicapped children.

TITLE OF ARTICLE: *The Nature of Interaction between Nursing Staff and Profoundly Multiply Handicapped Children*

Main research question What is the rate, content and appropriateness of interaction between staff and profoundly mentally handicapped children?

Research design and method Ten children aged between 10 and 22 years were observed in a ward in a large mental handicap hospital for a total of 10 hours and a detailed observational record was kept of the children's behaviour and of any related staff reactions.

Main findings There was little in the way of organised constructive activity and the children spent most of their time doing nothing. Staff attention appeared to be arbitrary and indiscriminate. Positive responses were more common than negative responses. However, there was no evidence of systematic strategies aimed at reinforcing desirable behaviour.

It was also found that interaction levels between staff and children were very low, and 83.7% of the children's behaviour which could have become the basis of a nurse–child interaction occurred in the absence of a nurse.

Implications This study of nurse–child interaction patterns is of crucial importance, and has implications for all age groups of residents with a mental handicap. It is often claimed that mental handicap nurses have rejected more 'traditional' nursing activities related to clinical procedures in favour of developing 'higher level' interpersonal, communication and teaching skills. Yet the previous studies cast doubts upon the validity of such assertions.

There is little point in carrying out elaborate assessment procedures with a person if such assessment does not become a basis for nursing action. Terms such as 'creating a stimulating environment' and 'helping a person to maximise their potential' become glib cliches in the absence of good quality interactions between the nurse and resident. However, effecting changes in nurses' work patterns can be very difficult.

Attempts have been made to implement staff training programmes in behavioural and communication techniques but this alone seems unable to overcome the powerful influence of the hospital as an institution with all of its constraints, as described in the studies of Shaw and Heyman (1982) and Alaszewski (1986). Beail's study points clearly to the need for much more research in the area of improving interaction between mental handicap nurses and the people they care for.

Rawlings (1985) found that by implementing changes in ward management practices, the quality of interactions could be improved. When staff were given more autonomy and responsibility, and when they were determined to allow residents to do as much for themselves as possible, then the residents' level of 'engaged activity' was higher. Rawlings (1985) concluded that it was possible, even within a rigidly run institution, for the residents' daily lives to be improved to an appreciable extent.

Techniques of 'room management' have also been used successfully to raise residents' activity levels (Sturmey et al. 1983; Partridge et al. 1985). Using this technique, one nurse is responsible for maintaining high levels of activity and contact while another nurse functions as the 'helper'. Wood (1985) describes room management activity sessions for mentally handicapped adults in long-stay hospitals and claims that these sessions increase team cohesiveness amongst the staff.

Community care

Community care has been viewed by most workers concerned with people who have mental handicaps as being universally desirable. However, the term 'community care' is so nebulous that few people can be certain as to what it really means. Moreover, there have been few attempts to examine the reality behind the rhetoric for people with mental handicaps and their families.

In a study of families in North Humberside, Ayer (1984a, 1984b) and Ayer and Alaszewski (1984) examined how families who had a child with a severe mental handicap saw this concept of 'community care'.

TITLE OF BOOK: *Community Care and the Mentally Handicapped: Services for Mothers and their Mentally Handicapped Children*

Main research questions   How do mothers describe the process of bringing up a handicapped child at home?

Research method and design   Over a 3-year period the researcher interviewed 132 mothers whose children were all aged between 3 and 17 years and attending special schools in the area. An open-ended interviewing schedule was used.

Mothers were the subjects of the interviews, as it is women within families who usually have the responsibility for providing the bulk of daily care for the child who has a handicap. Discussion of the various topics gave the mothers the chance to describe the reality of caring for a child with a mental handicap at home 'in the community'. The researcher asked the mothers to describe several aspects of their lives caring for a handicapped child. In particular, they were asked about the problems they experienced in carrying out the child's daily care, the assistance they received and from whom, their perceptions of their child's handicap and the kind of informal and formal support the mothers received from family and social services.

Main findings   Ayer (1984a) summarised the findings of this study as being an example of the failure of professionals to meet family needs. Mothers were critical of almost every aspect of professional involvement – or the lack of it. The lives of many of these mothers were described as ones of 'unrelenting daily grind' as they tried with minimal support to cope with the increasingly difficult tasks related to the daily physical care of their children. Incontinence was cited as a major problem.

Generally, mothers had little knowledge of support services and facilities which were available. Ayer uses Spitzer's (1975) terms to describe how social and community services viewed the needs of such families. Unlike 'social dynamite' problems, e.g. drug abuse, child abuse and family violence, where a newsworthy threat is posed, these mothers of handicapped children were considered to be 'social junk' whose problems were undramatic and created a burden only in economic terms.

The mothers were asked to say how useful various care professionals had been. It was found that the majority of mothers did not see social workers or health visitors as either helpful or well informed and would have preferred regular visits from an interested specialist. Ayer & Alaszewski (1984) and Ayer (1984b) concluded that without exception, the families were willing and determined to carry out primary care. However, they required services which supported and reinforced their attempts to care for their own children, not alternative services that replaced their efforts.

Implications This study demonstrates that for many families caring for a person with a mental handicap, 'community care' is more of a myth than a reality – something which exists in policy documents but which bears little relation to their daily lives.

Community care staff can draw little comfort from this study. It seems that providers of services have failed to find out from the families themselves the kinds of services that they feel would be valuable. At present consumers find that provision of support tends to be ad hoc and crisis oriented (Ayer 1984a). This is an area which clearly merits further research.

It seems likely, however, that improvements in the care of people with mental handicaps will not come about as a result of simply altering working procedures. What is needed is a shift in nurses' perceptions of both their role and of the very nature of the people with whom they work. Many would argue that such a re-evaluation should be based upon the principle of normalisation (The Campaign for People with Mental Handicaps 1981).

This approach was first developed in the mid 1970s and has been incorporated as part of the development of the All Wales Strategy (AWS) attempt to provide a truly integrated and comprehensive service (Grant 1985; Evans *et al.* 1986). Implementing change on such a large scale is naturally difficult but initial evaluations of the AWS have been promising as some studies (Allen & Donovan 1986; Donovan & Allen 1986) have shown.

This approach is based upon the positive valuing of people with mental handicaps and on maintaining a clear focus upon the quality and variety of environment and experiences available. This represents a basis for the planning and provision of nursing services which may ensure that nurses could justifiably consider themselves to be the key staff involved in the care of people with mental handicaps, especially in mental handicap hospitals. Nurses can no longer claim to enjoy this special relationship simply by virtue of being 'in contact' with the person for a longer period than others.

Summary and suggestions for further research

There is a need for many more mental handicap nurses to begin to undertake research for themselves into the problems and issues which concern them and those they care for. At the same time, much can be gained by looking to other disciplines, such as education and psychology, to provide some of the theoretical basis for nursing practice.

However, in conjunction with this need for increased research involvement on the part of mental handicap nurses, there is a need for a widening of the research perspective within mental handicap. While the traditional emphasis upon behavioural and experimental types of research has produced work which nurses have found to be valuable, the preponderance of this approach has tended to obscure the need for what might be termed more qualitative studies.

There is a strong tradition of excellent qualitative work in the field of mental handicap in, for example, the work of Oswin (1978), Bogdan *et al.* (1974), Bogdan and Taylor (1975) and Cleland (1979). A further shift in research emphasis towards more qualitative methods could begin to redress the rather arrogant assumptions which professionals occasionally make whereby they 'understand' the mentally handicapped person's needs and desires and 'know' what services are wanted or required without actually consulting mentally handicapped people themselves or trying to gain some understanding of their world.

The changes which have occurred in mental handicap over the past 20 years have placed an increased emphasis upon the nature of mentally handicapped people as people in their own right rather than as a collection of 'clinical features' or a human manifestation of a gamut of 'problems'. Such a 'person-centred' perspective is similar to the perspective of the qualitative researcher who will generally be attempting to describe, or understand, the problems or phenomena from the 'native's' point of view, i.e. the nurse, the mentally handicapped person or the family.

The move towards community care has gained momentum

over the past 20 years but it could be argued that this momentum has been driven by professionals who have tended to define the needs of families without paying sufficient attention to the views of the families themselves. Since the early 1970s there have been major changes in the patterns of care provided for people with mental handicaps. Such changes have had profound implications for mental handicap nurses, for they have had to re-examine radically almost every aspect of their role and, indeed, the concept of 'mental handicap' itself. However, in general this process of critical self-examination has been carried out in a spirit of defensiveness rather than with professional self-confidence. Mental handicap nurses have devoted considerable energies to discussing and researching questions and issues related to the future of mental handicap nursing, such as 'who should care for the mentally handicapped?'. As Tierney (1983) has noted, it is unfortunate that such preoccupation with intraprofessional introspection has deflected nurses' attention from urgent questions related to the needs of people with mental handicaps and their families and how well these are being met.

It could be argued that developments in mental handicap in the last decade have been occurring with greater frequency and diversity than in other areas of nursing. Community care, advocacy, integration, normalisation and many other ideas have challenged the traditional practices of mental handicap nurses and the need for continuing research in all these areas is great.

References

Alaszewski A. (1986) *Institutional Care and the Mentally Handicapped – The Mental Handicap Hospital*. London: Croom Helm

Allan E. & Goodbody L. (1984) Staff pay hardly any attention to mentally handicapped patients. *Nursing Mirror*, **158**, 17, 10

Allen D. & Donovan T. (1986) The AWS from a parent's point of view: Part 2 – Services' use and consumer satisfaction. *Mental Handicap*, **14**, 2, 71–74

Ayer S. (1984a) Community care: Failure of professionals to meet family needs. *Child: Care, Health and Development*, **10**, 127–140

Ayer S. (1984b) Handicapped children in the community. *Nursing Times* Occasional paper, **80**, 117, 66–69

Ayer S. & Alaszewski A. (1984) *Community Care and the Mentally*

Handicapped: Services for Mothers and their Mentally Handicapped Children. London: Croom Helm

Beail N. (1985) The nature of interactions between nursing staff and profoundly multiply handicapped children. *Child: Care, Health and Development*, **11**, 3, 113–129

Blackwell M.W. (1979) *Care of the Mentally Retarded.* Boston: Little, Brown & Co

Bogdan R. & Taylor S. (1975) This is their home. In Bogdan R. & Taylor S. (Eds) *Introduction to Qualitative Research Methods.* Chichester: John Wiley & Sons

Bogdan R., Taylor S., De Grandpre B. & Haynes S. (1974) Let them eat programs: attendants' perspectives and programming in wards in state schools. *Journal of Health and Social Behaviour*, **15**, 142–151

The Campaign for People with Mental Handicaps (1981) *The Principle of Normalisation: A Foundation for Effective Services.* (Available from CMH, 12a Madox Street, London, W1R 9PL.)

Cleland C.C. (1979) *The Profoundly Mentally Retarded.* Englewood Cliffs, New Jersey: Prentice-Hall

Cullen C., Burton M., Watts S. & Thomas M. (1983) A preliminary report on the nature of interactions in a mental handicap institution. *Behaviour Research and Therapy*, **21**, 5, 579–583

Donovan T. & Allen D. (1986) The AWS from a parent's point of view: Part 1 – Attitudes towards integrated services. *Mental Handicap*, **14**, 1, 19–21

Evans G., Beyer S., Todd S. & Blunden R. (1986) Planning for the All Wales Strategy. *Mental Handicap*, **14**, 3, 108–110

Felce D., Mair T., de Kock U., Saxby H. & Repp A. (1985) An ecological comparison of small community based houses and traditional institutions – II. Physical setting and the use of opportunities. *Behaviour Research and Therapy*, **23**, 3, 337–348

Grant G. (1985) Towards participation in the All Wales Strategy: Issues and processes. *Mental Handicap*, **13**, 2, 51–54

Oswin M. (1978) *Children in Long Stay Hospitals.* London: Heinemann/SIMP

Partridge J., Chisholm N. & Levy B. (1985) Generalisation and maintenance of ward programmes: Some thoughts on organisational factors. *Mental Handicap*, **13**, 1, 26–29

Paton X. & Petrusev B. (1974) The stimulation of verbal skills in the high grade mentally retarded patient: a nurse administered treatment procedure. *International Journal of Nursing Studies*, **11**, 2, 119–126

Rawlings S.A. (1985) Life styles of severely retarded non-communicating adults in hospitals and small residential homes. *British Journal of Social Work*, **15**, 281–293

Shaw M. & Heyman B. (1982) Changes in patterns of care of the

58 FURTHER RESEARCH FOR NURSING

mentally handicapped: Implications for nurses' perceptions of their
roles and hospital decision making processes. *Journal of Advanced
Nursing*, **7**, 555–563

Spitzer S. (1975) Towards a Marxian theory of deviance. *Social Problems*, **2**, 638–651

Sturmey P., Crisp T. & Dearden B. (1983) Room management with
profoundly handicapped young adults. *Mental Handicap*, **11**, 3,
118–119

Tierney A. (1973) Toilet training. *Nursing Times*, **69**, 1740–1745

Tierney A.J. (1983) *Nurses and the Mentally Handicapped*. Chichester:
John Wiley & Sons

Wood J.R.A. (1985) Room management activity sessions for adults
in long stay hospitals: Implications for staff and residents. *Mental
Handicap*, **13**, 2, 76–77

Chapter 6

The Care of Sick Children

DONNA M. MEAD

Hospitalisation and all that it entails can be a very difficult experience for children. Not only are they removed from the security of their own homes and separated from family and friends, but they also find themselves in an unfamiliar and sometimes threatening environment. They are confronted by strangers, and may have contact with as many as 25 different people within a 3-hour period (Lindheim *et al.* 1972) They have to sleep in a strange bed and eat strange food. They may not have their own familiar and much-loved toys with them and, in addition, they are likely to see and hear other children who are ill and in pain. They may have to undergo medical procedures which can hurt and confuse them. In short, nothing is normal or routine for a child or parent who has not been in hospital before.

The emotional effects of hospitalisation on children have been well documented. Much of the early research was concerned with the effects on the child of separation from the mother. Bowlby (1951) and Robertson (1956) describe how children between the ages of 6 months and 6 years who have been separated from their mother or primary care giver often react in a particular way. They outlined three stages through which the child passes. In the first stage of 'protest' the child cries loudly and angrily and refuses any attempt by others to get close to him and give care. The second stage is called 'despair', when the child is quiet and shows very little interest in anything. This stage was often mistakenly thought of as the 'settling-in stage'. It has led to much controversy about visiting, especially if when the mother arrives or leaves, the child cries and the mother is thus considered to have upset him. However,

Robertson (1970) showed that children tend to cry when their parents visit them only because it relaxes them enough to enable them to show feelings which have been bottled up. Finally there is a period called 'detachment', when the child appears to have accepted the situation, and this too has in the past often been thought to mean that the child has settled in. Robertson suggests that what is in fact happening is that the fear, sorrow and loneliness that the child has felt are repressed and the child begins to show more interest in his ward surroundings. At this stage, when the mother visits, the child no longer cries when she leaves and appears more interested in the sweets and gifts which she brings.

As a result of the work of these early researchers, the Platt Report (Ministry of Health 1959) recognised that children should be treated very differently from adult patients, and that particular attention should be paid to the emotional and mental needs of the child. One of the principal recommendations of the Platt Report was for the provision of facilities in children's wards so that the mothers could remain with their children throughout their stay. Whereas many hospitals now allow 24-hour visiting and have facilities for parents to stay, there is evidence to suggest that the recommendations of this report are not easily accepted by all nurses working in paediatric areas. In 1980, the Consumers Association study of over 50 hospitals found that only half of the hospitals in their sample had unrestricted visiting. The study also uncovered many other restrictions, such as no visiting during doctors' ward rounds, no visiting before 10 a.m., and no visiting at lunch or rest time. Harris (1986) found that many of the proponents of restricted visiting were the ward sisters. Poster (1983) notes that while many hospitals have instituted liberal visiting hours and rooming-in facilities in principle, often these policies do not reflect the reality of what is taking place.

Hawthorn (1974) observed that large numbers of nurses participated in the care of each child and that children in hospital spend a good deal of time alone. Rodin (1983) reports a description of a child who had 23 complete changes in staff during her stay in an orthopaedic hospital. These findings highlight the importance of patient allocation and primary nursing in paediatric units.

Research which followed that of Bowlby and Robertson

concentrated on the effect on the child of the parents' presence in hospital (Brain & Maclay 1968; Mahaffy 1965). These researchers found that the benefits of a parent's presence are psychological and physiological. Mahaffy (1965) has shown that the beneficial physiological effects of the mother's presence after tonsillectomy included a decreased incidence of vomiting and crying, a significant intake of fluids and a more speedy recovery than children in the control group. The results of the Brain and Maclay (1968) study of children admitted for tonsillectomy also showed a significant reduction in the incidence of emotional and infective complications when children were accompanied by their mothers.

Reactions to hospitalisation, however, vary from age to age. Whereas the pre-school child is most affected by separation from his parents, particularly his mother, children aged 5–11 years can increasingly tolerate separation from their parents, and the focus of anxiety shifts to fear of pain from injections or incisions and fantasies of mutilation. At puberty the focus of concern is likely to shift yet again towards fear of loss of personal control and the threat to their 'normality'.

Klinzing and Klinzing (1977) note that the primary reason for children's fear is a lack of understanding of the medical procedures, especially when no explanation or preparation is given to them. As a result children can create disturbing fantasies about what is involved with such procedures. For example, Moss (1981) noted that young children tend to perceive pain even in painless procedures such as having their blood pressure taken. The fantasy created in the absence of previous experience to predict what the procedure is like was thought to be more frightening than the procedure itself.

It can be seen, therefore, that as well as emotional support of the sort outlined above (i.e. presence of mother/primary care giver) children need factual information about what is involved with procedures. This was the concern of Rodin (1983), who stressed that the ignorance of hospitals and what goes on in them is another important contributory factor to the child's distress. The whole issue of preparing children and their parents for hospitalisation became the basis for Rodin's study.

There is general consensus that children should be prepared for an admission to hospital and to undergo the procedures, painful or otherwise, which are involved (Pinkerton 1980; Moss

1981; Visintainer & Wolfer 1975). It is usually agreed that children need and are eager to know what is going to happen to them, that they need to be forewarned and that they expect honesty and will become very unco-operative if any part of the procedure is different from that which was explained to them.

The problem which professionals have encountered, however, is one of deciding how to communicate such explanations effectively to the child and the parent. Children perceive the world differently from adults. This is reflected quite clearly in their communication behaviours, through thought, language and play. Therefore, any means of providing this factual information has to be adapted to suit a child's level of understanding and intellectual ability. Rodin (1983) considered that preparation for hospital, therefore, called for a variation in technique and management which would reflect the child's maturity and the circumstances of the admission, i.e. planned or emergency. In a comprehensive study she examined the ways in which children could be prepared for their experience in hospital.

A survey was undertaken from a wide cross-section of the population to establish their views about whether children aged 4–7 should be told about hospital, what they should be told, who should be responsible for telling them, and when this information should be given. The questionnaire was sent out to selected groups of parents, paediatricians, paediatric nurses, teachers, play group leaders and health visitors. There were many interesting findings and the reader is referred to Rodin (1983) for specific details. In summary, however, Rodin found that the responding groups said very clearly that all children aged 4–7 should be prepared for hospital and that such preparation should preferably be given as part of their general education. It was felt that more attention should be given to the subject by schools and the media and that there should be greater liaison between schools and hospitals.

Parents were identified as the most important group to tell children about hospital, but it was also felt that it was essential that simple and effective educational material be produced in order to help parents do this. It was considered important that children should always be told the truth.

Rodin (1983) subsequently undertook a specific research

project to examine the impact of the use of games to prepare children for investigations and procedures in hospital.

TITLE OF BOOK: *Will This Hurt?*

Main research question What effect will truthful preparation games have on the anxiety levels of hospitalised children undergoing a venepuncture procedure?

Research method and design The researcher spent about 50 2–3-hour sessions observing children's reactions to stress while undergoing various medical procedures in order to establish which medical procedure would produce the most suitable conditions in which to use preparation games. Selection criteria were that children should be aged 4–7 years; that they should be undergoing the procedure for the first time; and that they should have a parent to accompany them throughout the whole of the procedure. Venepuncture was identified as the most suitable procedure. The next step involved designing simple and truthful preparation games for venepuncture. The games had to be self-explanatory so that there would be no need for the involvement of professional staff and the games had to be suitable for parent and child to use together. Three games were produced: one was a colourful, cartoon-style activity book; the second a sorting board jigsaw; the third was an illustrated story book which could either be folded up concertina-style and then read page by page or could be opened out to form a wall frieze.

The preparation games were tested using a random sample of children who were involved in an EEC lead-level survey and who were having blood samples taken by venepuncture for this purpose. The selected children were randomly allocated to three groups. Group A children were provided with medical preparation games before having their blood test; they were quite free to play with them as they wanted and for as long as they wanted. Parents were asked to join in the play if they wished. Group B children were given ordinary games and Mr Man books with no medical content to play with. Group C children were given no games at all. The children's anxiety levels were measured by skilled phlebotomists on a 1–5 scale. The phlebotomists did not know which of the groups the children had been allocated to.

Main findings The results showed clear differences between the observed behaviour of Group A children and those of Groups B and C: Group A children exhibited more anxiety before the venepuncture but less during the procedure than children from Groups B and C. However, the anxiety of Group B and C children increased during the venepuncture beyond that of Group A children beforehand. Rodin concludes that the heightened anxiety of Group A children beforehand can be attributed to the fact that these children had come to realise something of what was going to happen to them.

The researcher was able to demonstrate three important points following analysis of the results. First, the material specially prepared for the preparation of children for the medical procedure of venepuncture was effective in reducing the anxieties of the children who had used the material during the blood test procedure, whereas the anxieties of children who had played with other material, or none at all, were found to rise at the time of the venepuncture. Second, the effectiveness of the material was appreciably increased if the children had been told beforehand about the blood test by their parents. Third, the anxiety shown by the children was clearly and directly related to the anxiety shown by the parents.

Implications Rodin concluded that if parents are informed and have been prepared about the medical procedures and about hospital, their children are more likely to be told and prepared and their anxiety will be lessened. The medical material which was specially prepared was effective for this purpose and could be used in the preparation of both children and parents before the procedure. The findings of this study do suggest that material giving information about hospital should be more extensively produced and distributed to parents. It is also clear that much further research is indicated into the experiences of the parents of children in hospital, in particular to examine the relationship between the perceptions and anxieties of the parents and the child.

Pain, accidents and family stress

Other studies concerned with the communication patterns of children include a small study by Jerrett and Evans (1986) which addressed children's pain vocabulary. The authors carried out a descriptive study to examine how a group of school-age children viewed their pain. The purpose of the research was to demonstrate that children can describe pain and that they do possess a pain vocabulary.

A sample of 40 school-age children who were attending an out-patient clinic for an acute health problem was included in the research. Each child was given a piece of white paper and a set of coloured pens and was asked to 'draw a picture that shows pain'. Upon completion of the task each child was asked to talk about the drawing. By categorising the adjectives the children used according to the tool provided by Melzack and Torgerson (1971), the researchers were able to demonstrate that children do use effective and evaluative descriptions of pain as well as sensory. In general the children's pain word descriptors were quite graphic and included statements such as 'like mosquitoes poking around in your ears' and 'pain makes you feel like screaming'. The researchers also attempted to rank the pain words the children used in terms of intensity using the McGill Pain Questionnaire (Melzack 1975).

This research is considered to be an initial step towards demonstrating that children can describe pain and that they do possess a pain vocabulary. It is a study that should be repeated in the UK. Larger samples of children are necessary to demonstrate whether children's pain words are consistently reproducible. The value of this sort of research for practice is that diagnosis of specific illness could be made easier and pain relief more effective.

The commonest single cause of admission to hospital for children age 1–14 is an accident, and clearly any research project which attempts to illustrate ways in which the incidence of childhood accidents can be reduced is to be welcomed. Laidman (1987) investigated the health visitor's role in the prevention of accidents to children between antenatal and pre-school age. In this research the health visitors' opportunities, knowledge and skills for accident prevention were examined and the author concludes that health visitors should spearhead local preventive programmes on a variety of subjects within the field of child accident prevention. They could also directly influence the safety behaviour of their clients and their colleagues in other professions.

As well as being the most common cause of hospital admission, childhood accidents are a significant cause of handicap and often leave the child with a chronic illness which results in frequent admissions to hospital. In her study *Families in Stress*, Harrison (1977) focused her attention on children suffering from one of two long-term conditions, Perthe's disease and cystic fibrosis. Her specific concerns were the patterns of stress experienced by the parents of these children. Although both conditions are disabling, require periodic hospital care and produce intermittent stress episodes, they differ in severity and prognosis. As the author states, the course of Perthe's disease is highly predictable, as are the associated parental stress patterns, while the progress of cystic fibrosis and the stress associated with it is highly unpredictable. During the exploratory phase of her work, Harrison developed hypotheses from her data which were tested in the main study. A combination of methods was used for this research; they included the examination of records, interviews with parents and professional staff, and diaries kept by parents. The main findings from this study related to the measures which professionals can take to reduce predictable stress in a condition which runs a predictable course. A general model was developed which has relevance to any illness situation and associated stress. In the author's words: 'The model calls attention to probable stress points and to policy and practices which may alleviate distress in the person and families concerned and it is suggested that it can be used by professional staff and by patients and their relatives'. Its particular application to terminal illness situations is emphasised. The implications of the availability of such a tool for practising nurses are obvious.

Summary

Until recently, paediatric nursing research in the UK concentrated predominantly on how children appear to feel when admitted to hospital and how they may be affected by the presence or absence of the mother or primary care giver. Such research, which has mainly involved observation techniques, has made a valuable contribution to the literature. It is equally important, however, that we hear from the children themselves how they feel, both physically and psychologically.

The problem is that in order to address this issue, researchers will first have to overcome the methodological difficulties inherent when communicating with children. This adds to the challenge of paediatric nursing research, as the researcher must use creativity and ingenuity in addition to conventional research skills in order to overcome the limitations in children's understanding that are associated with different stages of development.

Rodin's (1983) research is an example where an attempt has been made to respond to this challenge. Other ideas which have potential in future research include game techniques. For example, Brown (1985) used a 'three wishes' technique in her study to investigate children's understanding of diabetes, and Porter (1974) used body outline drawings to establish school-age children's perceptions and understanding of internal body structures. These ideas have exciting potential for future research, especially that which attempts to explore and address possible changes in a child's body image as a result of illness.

Another research approach which may prove valuable in the study of the nursing care of children is the use of the repertory grid technique. This technique has already been used to explore the subjective world of children who are deaf, mentally handicapped and who have behavioural problems (Baillie–Grohman 1975; Barton *et al*. 1976; Butler 1985). This approach helps to overcome inherent communication difficulties and the technique has been developed to incorporate the use of pictures, 'imagine that' scenes and mime in a most successful way (Ravenette 1975; Honess 1977; Baillie–Grohman 1975). The repertory grid technique could also be used to assess the way in which asthmatic children see their world and to investigate whether this view of their world can be changed as a result of participating in an exercise or education programme.

It is essential that nurse researchers in the field of paediatrics continue to develop methods appropriate for the participation of children. Games and make-believe have already been successfully used. Such approaches should be further exploited and others, such as story-telling, the use of toys and 'let's pretend', need to be developed. Just as the nursing care of children requires creativity, skill and knowledge, so it is essential that similar creativity skills and knowledge are integrated into paediatric nursing research.

References

Baillie-Grohman R.C. (1975) The use of a modified form of repertory grid technique. In Fransella F. and Bannister D. (Eds) *A Manual for Repertory Grid Technique*. London: Academic Press

Barton E.S., Walton J. & Rowe D. (1976) Using grid technique with the mentally handicapped. In Slater P. (Ed.) *Explorations of Personal Space*, Vol. 1. Chichester: John Wiley & Sons

Bowlby J. (1951) *Maternal Care and Mental Health*. Geneva: World Health Organisation

Brain D.T. & Maclay I. (1968) Controlled study of mothers and children in hospital. *British Medical Journal*, **1**, 603–608

Brown A.J. (1985) School age children with diabetes: knowledge and management of the disease and adequacy of self-concept. *Maternal Child Health Journal*, **14**, 1, 47–61

Butler R.C. (1985) Towards an understanding of children's difficulties. In Beail N. (Ed.) *Repertory Grid Techniques and Personal Constructs. Applications in Clinical and Educational Settings*. London: Croom Helm

Consumers Association (1980) *Children in Hospital*. London: Consumers Association

Harris P.J. (1986) Children, their parents and hospital in Muller D.J., Harris P.J. and Wattley L. (Eds) *Nursing Children. Psychology Research and Practice*. London: Harper and Row

Harrison S. (1977) *Families in Stress: A Study of the Long Term Medical Treatment of Children and Parental Stress*. London: Royal College of Nursing

Hawthorn P.J. (1974) *Nurse, I Want My Mummy*. London: Royal College of Nursing

Honess T. (1976) Cognitive complexity and social prediction. *British Journal of Social and Clinical Psychology*, **15**, 23–31

Jerret M. & Evans K.E. (1986) Children's pain vocabulary. *Journal of Advanced Nursing*, **11**, 403–408

Klinzing D.R. & Klinzing D.G. (1977) *The Hospitalised Child: Communication Technique for Health Personnel*. Englewood Cliffs, New Jersey: Prentice-Hall

Laidman P. (1987) *The Health Visitor's Role in the Prevention of Accidents to Children between Ante-natal and Pre-school Age*. London: Health Education Authority

Lindheim R., Glaser H.H. & Coffin C. (1972) *Changing Hospital Environments for Children*. Harvard, Mass.: Harvard University Press

Mahaffy P.R. (1965) The effects of hospitalisation on children admitted for tonsillectomy and adenoidectomy. *Nursing Research*, **14**, 12–19

Melzack R. (1975) The McGill Pain Questionnaire: major properties and scoring methods. *Pain*, **1**, 277–299

Melzack R. & Torgerson W.S. (1971) On the language of pain. *Anaesthesiology*, **34**, 50–59

Ministry of Health (1959) *Report of the Committee on the Welfare of Children in Hospital*. (Chairman: Sir Harry Platt). London: HMSO

Moss J.R. (1981) Helping your children to cope with the physical examination. *Paediatric Nursing*, **7**, 17–20

Pinkerton P. (1980) Preparing children for surgery. *On Call*, 5th June, 8–9

Porter C.S. (1974) Grade school children's perceptions of their internal body parts. *Nursing Research*, **23**, 5, 384–391

Poster E.C. (1983) Stress immunisation: Techniques to help children cope with hospitalisation. *Maternal Child Nursing Journal*, **12**, 119–134

Ravenette A.T. (1975) Grid techniques for children. *Journal of Child Psychology and Psychiatry*, **16**, 79–83

Robertson J. (1956) A mother's observations on the tonsillectomy of her four year old daughter (with comments by Anna Freud). *The Psychoanalytic Study of the Child*, **11**, 410–433

Robertson J. (1970) *Young Children in Hospital*. London: Tavistock

Rodin J. (1983) *Will This Hurt? Preparing Children for Hospital and Medical Procedures*. London: Royal College of Nursing

Visintainer M.A. & Wolfer J.A. (1975) Psychological preparation for surgical paediatric patients: the effect on children's and parents' stress responses and adjustment. *Paediatrics*, **56**, 187–202

Chapter 7

Midwifery Research

Tricia Murphy-Black

There has been a considerable increase in research published by midwives since the late 1970s. The funding for this research has been from a variety of sources, ranging from locally funded projects to Department of Health and Scottish Home and Health Department training fellowships, commissioned projects by the Health Education Authority, and grants for projects led by midwives as well as the annual Royal College of Midwives/Maws Research Scholarship. Dissemination of research has been helped by the regular Research and the Midwife conferences. This chapter gives some examples of research published by midwives in the UK, with more details of the major DHSS-funded project on the role and responsibilities of the midwife.

Antenatal care

A descriptive study by Methven (1982) documented the practice of the antenatal booking interview in hospital. She demonstrated that midwives merely recorded an obstetric history but, with a nursing process framework, a more complete and personal history could be obtained and used as a basis for a care plan to be followed throughout the pregnancy. The implementation of the nursing process in a maternity hospital has been evaluated (Adams *et al.* 1981; Bryar & Strong 1983; Bryar 1985). A retrospective study of the case notes of women attending a teaching midwives clinic within a maternity unit (Thomson 1984) investigated the outcome of childbirth. The aim of the teaching clinic is to teach student midwives normal midwifery. Of the 142 women studied, there was a majority of lower socio-economic group, single-parent families with high unemployment and a relatively large number of primigravidae. As 55% of the women were referred back to the obstetricians, it was questioned whether they were suitable for a teaching clinic and suggested that there should be a separate midwives' clinic for this group of women.

Health education

A survey of 153 pregnant women to determine their knowledge of the suitability of dried milks for babies by Watson and Morrison (1979) demonstrated nearly 40% were unaware of the differences between modified and unmodified milks. Black (1984) has shown that only 9% of 143 mothers who smoked had stopped smoking during pregnancy, and that those who did so were moderate smokers only. Gillett (1976) reported that the preparation for childbirth classes she investigated were a great help to expectant mothers and fathers; this may, however, reflect the positive response invited in the question-naire used. The attendance of social classes four and five at antenatal classes was examined by Boswell (1979), who reported that timing and availability of transport were the major factors in deciding whether or not they would attend. One of Brammer's conclusions (1977) was that midwives were not sufficiently prepared for their role in antenatal education.

Labour and delivery

Perhaps the best known reports are the studies of the use of enemas and pre-delivery pubic shaving. Romney and Gordon (1981) showed that the incidence of faecal contamination, the length of labour and the number of babies with evidence of infection were similar in mothers who did and did not have an enema at the onset of labour; these results were supported by Drayton and Rees (1984). A recent preliminary report (Garcia et al. 1986) involving a survey of 193 English Health Districts in 1984 noted that pre-labour bowel preparation was routine in 16% of consultant units. There was no difference in the inci-dence of infection in three groups of mothers who were completely shaved, partially shaved or not shaved before delivery (Romney 1981), and the 1984 survey reported that mothers were completely shaved in only 1% and partially shaved in 37% of consultant units in England (Garcia *et al.* 1986).

Two studies of the birthing chair produced different results. A descriptive study (Romney 1983) compared 200 mothers, half of whom delivered in bed and half on the birthing chair. The advantages of the chair were that it allowed for more accurate assessment of pelvic capacity, reduced the number of instrumental deliveries and the incidence of backache in mothers with a posterior position. A small increase in blood loss was reported but this, it was argued, could be due to the fact that estimates of blood loss are more accurate when blood is not absorbed into the bedclothes.

A random sample of 100 women attending an antenatal clinic were interviewed in the second and third trimesters of pregnancy to determine their views of and attitudes to natural childbirth. Of the women interviewed, 42% were positively interested in natural childbirth and would use facilities such as a birthing stool or an alternative position (to lying in bed) for delivery, if available (Griffiths & Hare 1985).

A further clinical study, the joint work of obstetricians and a midwife, examined the use of a birth chair for delivery (Stewart *et al.* 1983).

TITLE OF ARTICLE: *A Randomised Trial to Evaluate the use of a Birth Chair for Delivery*

Main research question   What are the benefits and hazards of delivery in a commercially produced delivery chair?

Research design and method   The study included 189 mothers, with a single fetus presenting by the head, whose labours commenced, either spontaneously or by induction, between 37 and 42 weeks gestation. These mothers were randomly allocated towards the end of the first stage of labour into one of two groups: (a) to deliver in the birth chair, or (b) to deliver in the conventional recumbent position. Outcome measures included details of labour, delivery, blood loss and condition of the baby at birth.

Main findings   The ages, heights, weights, parity, gestational ages and social classes of the mothers in the two groups were similar. There were 99 mothers allocated to the chair group and 90 who were allocated to the bed group. No statistical differences were found in the length of the second stage, the time spent bearing down, the number of operative deliveries, the mean birth weight or the condition of the baby at birth.

For primigravidae overall, there was no difference in the rate of forceps' use between the chair and bed groups. However the results suggested that the chair may have helped those primigravidae who had epidural analgesia to overcome the difficulties of delivering spontaneously, as a quarter of the number in the chair, compared with over half in the bed, required a forceps delivery for delay in the second stage. Of all those who delivered in the chair, there was a significantly higher mean blood loss at delivery in multigravidae and significantly fewer primigravidae had episiotomies or only superficial damage to the perineum.

Implications The recent trend in midwifery practice to allow mothers more choice during their labour has involved a variety of birth chairs, stools or bars to aid delivery, but this is the first published study of a randomised controlled trial. Although the element of choice for the mothers was removed once they had given their consent to inclusion in the study, and the labours were actively managed, there were no major advantages to delivering in a birth chair compared to the bed. The main disadvantage of increased bleeding postpartum could, in the authors' view, be explained by the greater number of rapid deliveries, the increase in the venous pressure around the perineum, and possibly the greater ease of collecting and therefore measuring the blood loss from delivery in the chair. The use of the chair allowed mothers to adopt a position which aided pushing yet gave access to both the perineum and the baby.

Pain relief The use of meptazinol for pain relief in labour was reported by Knights (1986). Although there were no publications of the routine use of this drug at the time of the trial, the report does not mention if the mothers were informed or if their consent was obtained. One hundred and thirty-three mothers, randomly selected, were given single or repeated doses by intramuscular injection. The analgesic efficacy for the mothers and the low incidence of side-effects in both mothers and babies suggested that meptazinol may have advantages over pethidine.

A study of 19 mothers reported the effects of transcutaneous electrical nerve stimulation (TENS). There were 8 who found it useful, in 7 it had no effect, 3 reported it useful only in early labour, and 1 mother did not like the sensations (Howie 1985). Beazley and Ward (1978) demonstrated a significant difference in the number and type of complaints of perineal discomfort from mothers who had epidural compared with other forms of analgesia in labour. Postnatally, the use of strong parenteral analgesics (such as pethidine) was of little proven value over the combined use of simpler oral analgesia and local counterirritant.

Episiotomy

A study of 1000 mothers, aimed at minimising perineal trauma and randomised them into two groups (Sleep *et al.* 1984). Where episiotomy was restricted to fetal indications, the rate was 10%; in the group where the use was more liberal to restrict perineal tears, the rate was 51%. There were no significant differences between the two groups in the incidence of maternal pain or urinary symptoms at 10 days and 3 months postpartum, nor were there any differences in neonatal outcome. The group with the restricted policy had a greater number with an intact perineum but were more likely to have perineal and labial tears and to have resumed sexual intercourse by 1 month after delivery. The authors felt there was little support for the liberal use of episiotomy, and that the use of episiotomy does not decrease postpartum morbidity. In a retrospective study, Wilkerson (1984) analysed the episiotomy rate of 21 midwifery sisters who conducted or supervised at least 50 deliveries in the year. The range of episiotomy rate per midwife was wide – from 6.1% to 67.3%. Although the majority who performed episiotomy most frequently did so both for primigravidae and multigravidae, some had a high rate for the former and a low rate for the later. In the mothers, the episiotomy rate ranged from 12.5% to 92.8% for primigravidae, and from 3.0% to 57.1% for multigravidae. By comparison, Wilkerson reported that the *lay* midwives delivering babies in a commune (the Farm, Tennessee) had an overall episiotomy rate of 20% and an intact perineum rate of 54%.

Information and support

In a study of women's views, of 200 women interviewed, those with electronic fetal monitoring (EFM) were more likely to report that they felt restricted in their movements than were those monitored by intermittent auscultation. The EFM group had an increase in the number of women who reported they were left alone for short periods (Garcia *et al*. 1984).

Kirkham (1983) reported on the difficulties women have in obtaining information while they are in labour. Women picked up cues from the staff around them and, if they were told nothing, felt they could not ask for the information they required. Midwives and mothers were involved in a study of the artificial rupture of membranes (ARM) which used both interviews and observations. The data indicated that midwives rupture the membranes without consulting the mother (Henderson 1984). The report concluded that midwives deceived themselves about the reasons for doing the ARM; they imagined they had more autonomy than they had and that the decisions were directly or indirectly influenced by the medical staff.

Caesarian section

The perception of birth was found to be significantly less positive in mothers who had an emergency caesarean section (CS) compared with those who had a spontaneous delivery (Kirchmeier 1984). As those whose CS was planned had a more positive perception of birth than those whose CS was unplanned, Kirchmeier recommended that mothers should be warned about the possibility of CS.

Two established customs – the wearing of face masks in the labour ward and the use of shoe size as an indicator of pelvic disproportion – have been challenged. The infection rate, determined by high vaginal and perineal swabs, was shown to be 7.5% when masks were not worn compared with 9.6% during a mask-wearing period (Hunter & Williams 1985). Frame *et al*. (1985) demonstrated that mothers with a shoe size below 4½ had a 21% CS rate; those with shoe sizes of 4½–6 had a 10% CS rate; while those with shoe sizes of 6½ or above had a 1% CS rate; but a similar relationship with height could not be established.

Postnatal care

Ball (1981) undertook a study of 178 mothers, classified as low risk at the beginning of pregnancy, who delivered in two consultant units and two GP units. Data were obtained from hospital and community midwives as well as from a questionnaire to the mothers between 6 and 8 weeks postpartum to evaluate perception of care and assess emotional state. There were significant differences at 6–8 weeks postpartum in the emotional state which were associated with levels of satisfaction with postnatal care, patterns of parentcraft teaching, mothers' attitudes to the baby at birth, and social class. In a subsequent study (Ball 1983), 278 mothers from three hospitals were interviewed at 36 weeks of pregnancy (to assess their personality); at 24–48 hours after delivery; and were sent a questionnaire at 6 weeks postpartum to measure emotional wellbeing and satisfaction with motherhood. Hospital and community midwives were asked to assess the mothers' progress and needs during the postnatal period. The findings supported the need for individualised care for the mothers to assist them in the transition to motherhood. A study of third-day blues, using Stein's 'blues' questionnaire, obtained data every day for a week from maternity, gynaecological, female surgical and male surgical patients, and showed the incidence of the blues was nearly 60% in all the female patients, and 20% in males (Levy 1984).

Of three methods of calming babies – intra-uterine sound, a musical box playing a nursery rhyme, and natural methods such as talking, rocking and patting – the intra-uterine sound was significantly more effective compared with a combination of the musical box and natural methods (Callis 1984).

A group of 11 student midwives (Fenton *et al.* 1985) surveyed 100 primiparae about the length of stay in hospital because of local conditions causing a shortage of beds. The average stay in 1982 was 3.9 days, compared with 10.2 days in 1962. During the study period in 1982, 11% of mothers would have liked to have stayed longer, whereas 46% would have preferred a shorter stay. While the majority of mothers were satisfied with their care, many felt they did not get enough support from the midwives in hospital.

A study of the postnatal examination focused on the uptake

rate of a random sample of 210 women, 190 of whom were interviewed at home. Postal questionnaires to 102 GPs had a response rate of 54%. There were 90% of primiparous and 86% of multiparous women who attended the postnatal examination. The highest rate of non-attendance was in the primiparous women who were unemployed, single or students. At 8–10 weeks postpartum, 46% of the sample were still experiencing a range of problems. The GPs reported a similar range of problems but rated episiotomy more frequently than the women. Of the female GPs, 80% discussed sexual relations while only 57% of the male GPs reported that they did. Forty-five per cent of the mothers would prefer a female to carry out the examination if given a choice (Bowers 1984).

Infant feeding

Maclean (1977) surveyed midwives and health visitors with two questionnaires about breast-feeding (response 62%) and artificial feeding (response 70%). There was evidence of lack of continuity of care which predisposed to widespread problems and conflicting advice. There was considerable variance in the views between both the midwives and health visitors. The hypothesis that fair-haired and red/auburn-haired mothers have more problems with breast-feeding than dark-haired mothers was tested in a survey of 600 mothers. A larger proportion of fair/red-haired and a smaller proportion of brown/dark-haired mothers bottle fed. There was no difference in the incidence of problems with feeding when hair colour was compared but there was an association with problems and first parity, as well as with forceps delivery compared with normal delivery (Brockway 1986). Support for breast feeders on a fortnightly basis for the duration of feeding in a group of 28 mothers was compared with a group who were not supported by a midwife (Houston 1984). There were significantly more supported mothers who continued to feed during the first 12 weeks and they gave supplementary food significantly later than the control group. Mothers in social classes two, three and four appeared to benefit most from the home visits.

Midwifery education

A survey of 906 newly qualified midwives who undertook the 12-month midwifery training in 1979 had a response rate of 78%. A subjective assessment of the adequacy of the training revealed that the three areas that midwives felt to be inadequate were home confinements, caring for babies in special care units, and teaching groups of parents. There was a fourth and smaller group who were not confident in caring for babies in the labour ward. The midwives felt there was not enough time spent on teaching by hospital midwives in the clinical setting. There were 77.2% who intended to practise for at least a short period after qualification (Golden 1980). When these results were compared with a similar survey of those who had the 18-month training (Robinson 1986), the midwives were more likely to undertake the longer training because they wanted to practise as midwives and more were likely to intend to make a career in midwifery. In Scotland, the opinions of the 18-month trained midwives were sought (Pope 1986) as well as those of the qualified midwives, a total of 2127 midwives with a 53% response rate. The newly qualified midwives expressed satisfaction with the training and the previously qualified midwives thought they were well prepared. The factors which needed closer examination were the clinical objectives and clinical teaching; preparation for management; the delegation of progressive responsibility; and the position of student midwives as RGNs undertaking a post-basic training programme. Mander (1983), in a descriptive study of student midwives, examined the characteristics of those who continued and those who discontinued their training. She felt that more career advice is needed to help nurses plan their careers and this advice should present a realistic picture of what midwives do and what midwifery involves.

The role of the midwife

Walker (1975) reported that, although midwives saw themselves as practitioners in their own right in the care of normal pregnancy, obstetricians saw them as nurses who assist obstetricians but who have little more decision-making delegated to them by doctors than other nurses. She went on to ask if recognition and acceptance of their responsibility would enable midwives to give a better service. Black *et al.* (1984) reported some confusion between midwives and health visitors as to their respective roles in antenatal education. The data suggest that both groups exhibit co-operation and conflict in describing their roles and those of their colleagues.

The DHSS commissioned a large study on the role and the responsibilities of the midwife (Robinson *et al.* 1983). The main instruments were questionnaires to provide data for descriptive analysis of many aspects of the midwives' role. A survey of nationally drawn samples from 60 health districts in England and Wales produced a response from 4248 midwives (78%), 1177 health visitors (89%), 1232 general practitioners on the obstetric list (67%), and 333 medical staff in obstetrics (55%). A subsample of 74 midwives from a wide range of situations was given a semi-structured taped interview.

The overlap between the roles of the midwives and medical staff in the provision of normal antenatal care found by Robinson *et al.* demonstrated considerable erosion of the midwives' role as well as a waste of financial and manpower resources. Although a large majority of midwives reported that they cared for women in normal labour, much of their freedom to use their own clinical judgement was restricted where the management of labour was determined by unit policy or a doctor. Community midwives undertook few, if any, home confinements, and it was the views of the medical staff which determined whether community midwives were able to book home confinements.

In postnatal care, the community midwives' responsibility did not overlap with medical staff and they made the decision that a mother was fit to be discharged from midwifery care, unlike the hospital midwives who rarely made the decision that mother and baby were fit for transfer to community care.

There were significant differences in the perceptions of midwives and medical staff as to who was responsible for the management of normal antenatal and intrapartum care, with doctors more likely than midwives to indicate that doctors were involved in antenatal assessment and managing normal labours. There were wide variations in the role fulfilled by midwives, with the midwives working in separate general practitioner units having the greatest responsibility. The degree of clinical responsibility of the community midwives was not related to attachment to a general practitioner but to the views of the general practitioners with whom they worked. Few midwives had opportunities to provide continuity of care from the start of the pregnancy to the end of the puerperium.

Summary

This research raises many important questions and issues about the present and potential role of the midwife, and these merit further investigation. Until recently, the midwifery profession has lagged behind the nursing profession in research but is now beginning to question and investigate all areas of its practice. The speed of dissemination and implementation of some research findings is encouraging. This has been associated with those practices which the childbearing women were also questioning. While response to consumer demand is welcomed, midwives need to be proactive rather than reactive so that they will be able to assure the women in their care that their practice is research based.

References

Adams M.E., Armstrong-Esther C., Bryar R., Duberley J., Strong G. & Ward E. (1981) Trial run – the nursing process in Midwifery. *Nursing Mirror*, **153**, 15, 32–35

Ball J.A. (1981) Effect of present patterns of maternity care on the emotional needs of mothers, Parts 1, 2 and 3. *Midwives Chronicle*, **94**, 150–154, 198–202, 231–233

Ball J.A. (1983) Moving forward in postnatal care: Some aspects of a research project. *Midwives Chronicle*, **93** (Suppl.), 14–16

Beazley J.M. & Ward J.P. (1978) Perineal pain after epidural analgesia in labour. *Midwives Chronicle*, **91**, 204–206

Black P.M. (1984) Who stops smoking in pregnancy? *Nursing Times*, **80**, 19, 59–61

Black T., Booth K. & Faulkner A. (1984) Co-operation or conflict? How midwives and health visitors view each other's contribution to antenatal education. *Senior Nurse*, **1**, 25–26

Boswell J. (1979) Are classes 4 and 5 paying attention? *Nursing Mirror*, **148**, 12, 24–25

82 FURTHER RESEARCH FOR NURSING

Bowers J. (1984) Is the six week postnatal examination necessary?
The Practitioner, **229**, 1113–1115

Brammer A.C. (1977) *Organised Classes for Pregnant Women and
their Partners in Preparation for Childbirth and Parenthood*. An
enquiry into the classes provided by the Maternity Services in
England in 1975. Maws Ed. Research Scholarship 1974/75. London:
Royal College of Midwives

Brockway L. (1986) Hair colour and problems in breast feeding.
Midwives Chronicle, **99**, 66–67

Bryar R. (1985) An assessment of the introduction of systematic individualised care into midwives practice. Paper presented to the RCN
Research Society Conference 1985

Bryar R. & Strong G. (1983) Trial run – continued. *Nursing Mirror*,
157, 15, 45–48

Callis P.M. (1984) The testing and comparison of the intra-uterine
sound against other methods for calming babies. *Midwives Chronicle*, **97**, 336–338

Drayton S. & Rees C. (1984) 'They know what they're doing': The
midwife and enemas. *Nursing Mirror*, **159** (5, Suppl.), iv–viii

Fenton J., Hartwell C., Jambaccus A., Lee S., Lees J., O'Neill P.,
Rainford D.J., Rawlinson K., Sweeney B. & Ward J. (1985) Length
of stay in hospital after delivery of a first baby. *Midwives Chronicle*,
98, 156–159

Frame S., Moore J., Peters A. & Hall D. (1985) Maternal height
and shoe size as predictors of pelvic disproportion: An assessment.
British Journal of Obstetrics and Gynaecology, **92**, 1239–1245

Garcia J., Garforth S. & Ayres S. (1986) *The Policy and Practice in
Midwifery Study: Progress Report*. MIDIRS Information Pack No. 2

Garcia J., Corry M., MacDonald D., Elbourne D. & Grant A. (1984)
Mothers' view of continuous electronic fetal heart monitoring and
intermittent auscultation in a randomized controlled trial. *Research
and the Midwife Conference Proceedings*, 51–67

Gillett J. (1976) A report on the survey on preparation for childbirth
within the catchment area of Copthorne Maternity Unit, Shrewsbury: December 1972–June 1973. *International Journal of Nursing
Studies*, **13**, 25–46

Golden J. (1980) Midwifery training: The views of newly qualified
midwives. *Midwives Chronicle*, **93**, 190–194

Griffiths R. & Hare M.J. (1985) Do women really want natural childbirth? *Midwives Chronicle*, **98**, 92–94

Henderson C. (1984) Influences and interactions surrounding the
midwife's decision to rupture the membranes. *Research and the
Midwife Conference Proceedings*, 68–85

Houston M.J. (1984) Supporting breast feeding at home. *Midwives
Chronicle*, **97**, 42–44

Howie R. (1985) Client controlled pain relief in childbirth. *Midwives Chronicle*, **98**, 294

Hunter M.A. & Williams D. (1985) Mask wearing in the labour ward. *Midwives Chronicle*, **98**, 12–13

Kirchmeier R. (1984) Influences on mother's reactions to Caesarean birth. *Research and the Midwife Conference Proceedings*, 86–101

Kirkham M.J. (1983) Labouring in the dark: Limitations on the giving of information to enable patients to orientate themselves to the likely events and time scale of labour. In Wilson-Barnett, J. (Ed.) *Nursing Research: Ten Studies in Patient Care*. Chichester: John Wiley & Sons

Knights J. (1986) Use of meptazinol in routine obstetric practice in a district hospital. *Midwives Chronicle*, **99**, 182–183

Levy V. (1984) The 'third day blues'. *Midwives Chronicle*, **97** (Suppl.), xiv–xv

Maclean D. (1977) An appraisal of the concepts of infant feeding and their application in practice. *Journal of Advanced Nursing*, **2**, 111–126

Mander R. (1983) Stop and consider: student midwife wastage in training. *Research and the Midwife Conference Proceedings*, 38–52

Methven R. (1982) The antenatal booking interview: Recording an obstetric history or relating to a mother-to-be? *Research and the Midwife Conference Proceedings*, Part 1, 63–76; Part 2, 77–95

Pope V.E. (1986) Midwifery training in Scotland: An opinion survey. *Midwives Chronicle*, **99**, 198–200

Robinson S. (1986) Career intentions of newly qualified midwives. *Midwifery*, **2**, 25–36

Robinson S., Golden J. & Bradley S. (1983) *A Study of the Role and Responsibilities of the Midwife. Nursing Education Research Unit Report No. 1*. London: King's College, University of London

Romney M.L. (1980) Predelivery shaving: an unjustified assault? *Journal of Obstetrics and Gynaecology*, **1**, 33–35

Romney M.L. (1983) Chair project. *Research and the Midwife Conference Proceedings*, 69–80

Romney M.L. & Gordon J. (1981) Is your enema really necessary? *British Medical Journal*, **282**, 1269

Sleep J., Grant A., Garcia J., Elbourne D., Spencer J. & Chalmers I. (1984) West Berkshire perineal management trial. *British Medical Journal*, **289**, 587–590

Stewart P., Hillan E. & Calder A. (1983) A randomised trial to evaluate the use of a birth chair for delivery. *Lancet*, **ii**, 1296–1298

Thomson A. (1984) Antenatal care: An examination of the midwife's contribution. *Research and the Midwife Conference Proceedings*, 135–162

Walker J.F. (1976) Midwife or obstetric nurse? Some perceptions of midwives and obstetricians of the role of the midwife. *Journal of Advanced Nursing*, **1**, 129–138

Watson M. & Morrison E.M. (1979) Health education and infant feeding – does mother know best? *Midwives Chronicle*, **92**, 220–221

Wilkerson V.A. (1984) The use of episiotomy in normal delivery. *Midwives Chronicle*, **97**, 106–110

Chapter 8

The Care of Patients and Clients in the Community

JENNIFER LITTLEWOOD

Three professional groups of nurses are concerned with the care of patients and clients in the community: district nurses, health visitors and community psychiatric nurses, collectively referred to as community nurses (Littlewood 1987). In this chapter, the focus is on research in the general area of community nursing, that is, the area which falls within the responsibilities of district nurses and health visitors. Although there are similarities between the work of the district nurse and the health visitor in relation to health promotion, there are also distinct differences between them in working arrangements and clinical responsibilities. Therefore, it was decided to summarise two pieces of research, one particularly relevant for district nurses and the other for health visitors.

The development of research in the field of community nursing has only recently gained momentum and, in line with research in other types of nursing, studies of *nurses* preceded those concerned with *nursing*. As a crude way of providing an overview, it is possible to identify four categories of studies.

1. **The roles, functions and deployment patterns of community nurses**. Early descriptive studies provided some of the impetus for further work. Hockey (1966) and Clark (1973) focused on the work of district nurses and health visitors respectively. Probably because of the identified problems and anomalies, many further studies were initiated. A useful summary of the health visitor's role and functions was undertaken by Clark (1981). Dunnell and Dobbs (1982) conducted a detailed survey of nursing staff working in the community, to establish who worked in the community and the types of

85

patients and clients they looked after. This followed earlier attempts by Hockey (1972) and by McIntosh and Richardson (1976), and used a similar design. Thus, some changes in staff composition and patient/client groups over time could be identified.

Deployment studies include detailed examinations of community nurses working in a variety of roles. Whilst the above study by Dunnell and Dobbs (1982) included treatment room/practice nurses, a 4-year prospective study of the nurse in the treatment room was undertaken by Waters *et al.* (1980) and, in the following year, two of the researchers involved in the study provided a detailed analysis of treatment room procedures. They concluded from their findings that many procedures undertaken were not normally included in the nurse's training programmes. These findings clearly have implications for nurse education. More recently, the work pattern of the 'nurse practitioner', as an innovation within district nursing, has attracted research interest. Stilwell conducted most of the research in this field (Stilwell 1982, 1982b). Stilwell's work is on-going and the papers cited represent a mixture of descriptive experience and the beginnings of research; they show how practical experience can stimulate research.

2. **Organisational aspects of community nursing**. The main studies falling under this heading relate to nurses working in teams within general medical practice. In an early classical study, Gilmore *et al.* (1974) described the working patterns of nursing teams, drawing attention to one of the main findings that team work does not happen merely by providing nurses and general practitioners with a common base. More clearly defined organisational patterns were explored in many later studies, comparing particularly the work of nursing staff attached to general practice with that of nursing staff with geographical responsibilities and with nurses employed by the general practitioners. Well-known examples are the studies by Reedy *et al.* (1976 and 1980), which elicited the views of nurses as well as describing their work in considerable detail. They established that there was no consensus of opinion about the type of organisational structure that was the most acceptable.

Another early study examined the work of a district

nursing sister attached to a general hospital (Hockey 1970). It was a quasi-experimental study designed to explore the possibility and the effects of discharging patients from surgical wards earlier than had been common practice.

The above study was a natural precursor to others looking particularly at the gaps between the hospital and community in terms of continuity of care. Roberts (1975) identified a number of deficits which could be guarded against and developed a valuable tool for nurses to aid continuity of care. The work by Skeet (1970) was based on interviews with patients and their relatives after discharge from hospital. It was presented in the form of case studies which, by the glaring problems revealed, attracted considerable publicity and generated further research in that area. Wilson-Barnett and Fordham (1982) suggested that lack of discharge planning is one of the factors responsible for delay in recovery at home. Communication problems between the hospital and community in the care of elderly patients were identified in a study by Melia and Macmillan (1983). Ross (1987) also focused attention on the lack of continuity of care.

Many other specific settings of community nursing practice are in need of systematic examination and description. They include the care of specific patient groups in the community, such as children and physically or mentally handicapped adults. Some references in other chapters of this book are relevant for community nurses also.

3. **Studies of clinical nursing problems**. Kratz (1978), in her study of the care of long-term patients by district nurses, demonstrated that such patients may be somewhat vulnerable because district nursing staff did not seem to 'value' them in the same way as they valued acutely ill patients or those making a recovery. The nurses had no clearly defined goal for such patients. Kratz's work made an important contribution in describing the situation as she found it, with scientific honesty.

Efforts to support the clinical work of community nurses by factual data are increasing. Most clinical nursing research is just as relevant to patients at home as to those in hospital. However, there are some clinical problems which feature prominently within the district nursing service. More than 20 years ago, Hockey (1966) highlighted the problem of leg ulcers by demonstrating the time-consuming nature of the care of patients with ulcers. Eighteen years later, Dale (1984) undertook a detailed survey among district nurses in two of Scotland's health board areas, which is described below.

TITLE OF ARTICLE: *Leg Work*

Main research questions   What are the demands of leg ulcer care on the National Health Service? What is the aetiology of leg ulcers? What are the healing and recurrence rates and what can be found out about compliance with treatment?

Research design and methods   Postal questionnaires were sent to appropriate health workers in order to locate patients with leg ulcers. Patients who gave their consent were then interviewed and examined, and in consequence information was collected from 600 patients. A random sample of high-risk group patients, aged 65 years or more, was investigated further.

Main findings   Only 7% of patients were less than 50 years old; district nurses cared for a high proportion of female elderly patients with leg ulcers. Leg ulcers heal slowly: 55% had been open for more than 6 months and 10% for more than 5 years. Two-thirds of the ulcers were recurrent. Many different treatments were in use; although compression is essential for the treatment of venous ulcers (Sigel *et al.* 1975), few bandages in current use are capable of producing adequate pressures.

Implications   The study has shown that the treatments used for leg ulcers are not always related to the type of ulcer. It is important for nurses to understand the aetiology of the condition and also to recognise the most vulnerable patient groups. For the effective treatment of venous ulcers, compression bandages should be used and crepe bandages are not suitable. The treatment of leg ulcers is costly and time consuming and further research in the form of clinical trials is necessary. In the meantime it would seem important to provide careful documentation for each patient treated.

Another study concerned with the problem of leg ulcers encountered by district nurses was undertaken by Nudds (1987). Its emphasis was on the giving of information to patients. The results suggested that patients' recovery can be aided by appropriately communicated and understood information. Other examples of clinical district nursing problems which have been studied are pain (Raiman 1986) and chronic wound care (Jones 1985). Both authors demonstrated the importance of assessing the whole patient within the home setting rather than focusing on the specific nursing problems in isolation. Ross studied self-medication by the elderly (Ross 1985, 1988) and constructed a drug guide to be used by this age group.

4. **Evaluative studies**. Evaluative studies denote the type of research question rather than the topic, and any area of health care can be evaluated.

An evaluative study in district nursing was undertaken by Illsley and Goldstone (1986). Entitled 'Measuring quality in district nursing', it took the form of a national survey. The predetermined quality criteria were the use of the nursing process, nursing records and models of nursing. Additional evaluative questions were asked. According to the authors, the survey has 'pulled together important and relevant information about the district nursing service which will influence the research and evaluation development of a quality evaluation tool . . .'

Two important studies under this heading tried to evaluate the work of the health visitor with the elderly. Luker (1982) compared the outcomes of specifically designed health visitor intervention with those of 'normal' health visiting, using individual client-specific goals. Vetter *et al.* (1984) measured effectiveness by a set of predetermined general outcomes, such as the ability to delay the rate of progression of physical, mental and social disability. Both studies used an experimental design and represented randomised controlled trials. Such a rigorous study design is necessary for objective evaluation (Holland 1983). The difficulties inherent in the application of such a design in real-life situations have been largely responsible for the slow development in evaluative work. Both the above studies demonstrated the potential of health visitor intervention with elderly persons.

It is of course, possible to evaluate services on the basis of predetermined goals. Thus if, for example, a slimming club is set up by health visitors and it is consistently well attended resulting in desired weight loss, it can be evaluated as effective. However, careful documentation is extremely important, especially for replication purposes. An example of such work is that of Wood and Alexander (1983), who demonstrated the positive effect of such a club for women.

The data for research need not always come from people directly; it is possible to undertake valuable studies based on written records, such as the study carried out by While (1986) which is summarised below.

TITLE OF ARTICLE: *The Uptake of Prophylactic Care During Infancy*

Main research question   What is the utilisation of the prophylactic child health services currently available within the National Health Service for infants during their first 24 months of life?

Research design and methods   Records were used as the main data sources. A questionnaire was designed to extract as much information as possible from health records in a systematic manner. Three types of record were used simultaneously: clinic record, home visiting record, and family record. The author defends the use of such records on the grounds of their reliability and rigourous completion.

The study took the form of a consensus and, therefore, no sampling technique was employed. A census means that all eligible study subjects are included in the study; in this instance, it included all infants resident in the selected geographical area on their second birthday. The area included inner city, suburban and affluent suburban homes. Interviews with health visitors yielded further data and also served the purpose of protecting confidential information from researcher access.

Main findings   Child health clinics were more frequently attended by the inner city infants than by those resident in suburbs. Uptake of developmental screening at 6 weeks was high in the three areas. Whilst uptake of immunisation was similar for the first dose, there was greater delay for the second dose in the suburbs than in the inner city. The third dose had lowest uptake rates. Highest uptake overall occurred in the inner city area. The same pattern was seen for measles immunisation, highest uptake rates being seen in the inner city. In contrast, hearing tests had highest attendance rates in the suburbs.

There was a positive association between employed people and uptake of services. Developmental assessments were less likely if the parents were dependent on supplementary benefits, in larger families, and if children who were bottle fed. Non-completion of the immunisation course was associated, amongst other things, with younger mothers, single parenthood and parental unemployment.

Implications The results of the study support many previous research findings concerning the provision and uptake of health care services. The researcher suggests that the value of the results for health visitors is that barriers to uptake of prophylactic care have been identified, that some families are vulnerable, and that there are clear associations between socio-economic status, mode of infant feeding practice and uptake of services. A thorough knowledge of the families, including an appreciation of their values and levels of understanding, may help health visitors to increase uptake of services.

Summary

The increase of research in community nursing, though accelerating, is slow in comparison with other fields of nursing. The emphasis on studies of role and functions and on organisational patterns is not surprising. The community nursing service is costly and it is important to identify effective structures for it and to gain greater clarity on role definitions and descriptions.

As in many other fields of health care, the search for quality assurance measures is on-going. For patients in the community, such measures are even more elusive because of the many uncontrollable variables in the home situation as compared with hospital. It is encouraging that an increasing number of nurses are trying to explore the clinical care they provide for their patients. Completed studies, especially those relating process to outcome, are beginning to show the contribution of community nurses to primary health care. It is hoped that this greatly condensed chapter illustrates the recent growth in research relevant to patients in the community. The impetus comes from many sources, important ones being the Declaration of Alma Ata (WHO 1978) and the Cumberlege Report (DHSS 1986).

In the vision of WHO, inherent in the Declaration of Alma

Ata (1978), of making health care accessible, available and acceptable to all by the year 2000, emphasis must be on care in the community. A dramatic extension of services, be they preventive, therapeutic or rehabilitative, without a sound foundation of research-based knowledge is, however, not likely to be in the best interest of either consumers or promoters, certainly not in the long term. Similarly, if the recommendations of the Cumberlege Report (DHSS 1986) are acted upon, much more research on the processes and implication of neighbourhood nursing will be urgently needed. Ross (1987) comments on the paucity of research in the area of consumer acceptability, and Bergman (1987) suggests that a master plan identifying priorities for community nursing research might be helpful.

If the emphasis on health teaching is to be expressed in practice rather than pure oratory, research needs to focus on matters such as health beliefs, attitude changes and cultural determinants of health behaviour.

Acknowledgement

I should like to thank Dr Lisbeth Hockey OBE for the considerable input, help and advice so kindly given during the preparation of this chapter.

References

Bergman R. (1987) Research in community nursing. In Littlewood J. (Ed.) *Community Nursing. Recent Advances in Nursing*. Edinburgh: Churchill Livingstone

Clark J. (1973) *A Family Visitor: A Descriptive Analysis of Health Visiting in Berkshire*. London: Royal College of Nursing

Clark J. (1981) *What do Health Visitors do? A Review of the Research 1960–1980*. London: Royal College of Nursing

Dale J (1984) Legwork. *Nursing Mirror*, **159**, 20, 22–25

Department of Health and Social Security (1986) *Neighbourhood Nursing – A Focus for Care. Report of the Community Nursing Review* (Chairman: J. Cumberlege). London: HMSO

Dunnell K. & Dobbs J. (1982) *Nurses Working in the Community: A Survey Carried out on Behalf of the DHSS in 1980*. London: HMSO

Gilmore M. *et al.* (1974) *The Work of the Nursing Team in General Practice*. London: Council for the Education and Training of Health Visitors

Hockey L. (1966) *Feeling the Pulse: A Study of District Nursing in Six Areas*. London: Queen's Institute of District Nursing

Hockey L. (1970) *Co-operation in Patient Care*. London: Queen's Institute of District Nursing

Hockey L. (1972) *Use or Abuse? A Study of the Enrolled Nurse in the District Nursing Service*. London: Queen's Institute of District Nursing

Holland W.W. (1983) *Evaluation of Health Care*. Oxford: Oxford Medical Publications

Illsley V. & Goldstone L. (1986) Measuring quality in district nursing. *Nursing Times*, **82**, 38–40

Jones K. (1985) Wound care in the community. *Journal of District Nursing*, **4**, 1, 4–5

Kratz C.R. (1978) *Care of the Long-Term Sick in the Community*. Edinburgh: Churchill Livingstone

Littlewood J. (1987) Community nursing – an overview. In Littlewood J. (Ed.) *Community Nursing. Recent Advances in Nursing*. Edinburgh: Churchill Livingstone

Luker K.A. (1982) *Evaluating Health Visiting Practice: an Experimental Study to Evaluate the Effects of Focused Health Visiting Intervention on Elderly Women Living Alone at Home*. London: Royal College of Nursing

McIntosh J.B. & Richardson I.M. (1976) *Work Study of District Nursing Staff*. Scottish Health Service Studies 37. Edinburgh: SHHD

Melia K.M. & Macmillan M.S. (1983) *Nurses and the Elderly in Hospital and the Community: A Study of Communication*. Edinburgh: Nursing Studies Research Unit, University of Manchester

Nudds L. (1987) Healing information. *Nursing Times Community Outlook*, September, 12–14

Raiman J. (1986) Monitoring pain at home. *Journal of District Nursing*, **4**, 11, 4–6

Reedy B.L.E.C. *et al.* (1976) Nurses and nursing in primary medical care in England. *British Medical Journal*, **2**, 1304–1306

Reedy B.L.E.C. *et al.* (1980) A comparison of activities and opinions of attached and employed nurses in general practice. *Journal of the Royal College of General Practitioners*, **217**, 483–489

Roberts I. (1975) *Discharged from Hospital*. London: Royal College of Nursing

Ross F. (1985) Uneasy bedfellows. *Nursing Times*, **81**, 44, 38–39

Ross F. (1987) District nursing. In Littlewood J. (Ed.) *Community Nursing. Recent Advances in Nursing*. Edinburgh: Churchill Livingstone

Ross F. (1988) Information sharing between patients, nurses and doctors: Evaluation of a drug guide for old people in primary health care. In Johnson R. (Ed.) *Excellence in Nursing. Recent Advances in Nursing.* Edinburgh: Churchill Livingstone

Sigel B., Edelstein A.L., Savage L., Hasty J.H. & Felix R. (1975) Type of compression for reducing venous stasis. *Archives of Surgery*, **110**, 171–175

Skeet M. (1970) *Home from Hospital: The Results of a Survey Conducted amongst Recently Discharged Patients.* London: Dan Mason Research Committee

Stilwell B. (1982a) The nurse practitioner at work. *Nursing Times*, **78**, 45, 1909–1910

Stilwell B. (1982b) The nurse practitioner at work. *Nursing Times*, **78**, 43, 1799–1803

Vetter N.J. *et al.* (1984) Effects of health visitors working with elderly patients in general practice. In While A. (Ed.) *Research in Preventive Community Nursing Care.* Chichester: John Wiley & Sons

Waters W.H., Sandeman J.M. & Lunn J. (1980) A four year prospective study of the practice nurse in the treatment room of a South Yorkshire practice. *British Medical Journal*, **280**, 87–89

While A. (1986) Uptake in prophylactic care during infancy. In While A. (Ed.) *Research in Preventive Community Nursing Care.* Chichester: John Wiley & Sons

Wilson-Barnett J. & Fordham F. (1982) *Recovery from Illness.* Chichester: John Wiley & Sons

Wood B. & Alexander E. (1983) Losing weight can be fun. *Nursing Mirror*, **156**, 11, 32–35

World Health Organisation (1978) *Primary Health Care: International Conference (Alma Ata).* Geneva: WHO

Part III: Research Issues in Nursing and Nursing Care

Introduction

JILL MACLEOD CLARK and LISBETH HOCKEY

Each of the six chapters in this section of the book addresses a professional issue or aspect of care which has relevance for nursing. Regardless of whether a nurse is working with the elderly or with premature babies, issues such as quality of care and interaction between nurses, patients and relatives are obviously of crucial importance. Similarly, clinical observations, pressure area care and patient teaching are aspects of care which are relevant to a wide range of nursing situations. The problem of manpower planning is one which continues to have a high profile, particularly whilst nurse managers have to battle for limited resources.

The authors of these chapters have attempted to present a concise picture of the research work that has been carried out in each area. In some cases, such as nurse–patient interaction and clinical observations, it does appear that we can lay claim to a developing body of knowledge, certainly at a descriptive level. In some other areas, notably that of patient teaching and pressure area care, the research is beginning to move towards measuring the outcomes of nursing interventions. However, it is perhaps issues such as manpower planning and quality of care which present the greatest professional challenge and where more research energy must be directed.

The material presented here just scratches the surface of what is available in these and many other areas of nursing. It is also clear that a great deal more research is required in all the areas addressed in this book, as well as in those we have not been able to include.

It is hoped the research described in these chapters will provide readers with many ideas for changing their practice,

give them much food for thought and provoke them into gener-
ating numerous new research questions.

Chapter 9

Clinical Observation

ROSAMUND HERBERT

Clinical observations are important monitors of a patient's physical condition and many clinical decisions are based on such observations. However, often observations seem to be a routine or ritual in nursing rather than a considered aspect of patient care. As a result they are not always made accurately or on the most appropriate occasions and so their value is reduced. Nurses carry out many different observations ranging from the so-called vital signs (temperature, pulse rate, respiratory rate, blood pressure), to neurological observations, fluid input and output, blood sugar levels, weight, peak flow and central venous pressure measurement. Most of the research in this area has looked at temperature and blood pressure measurements and this review will therefore concentrate on these observations. It is worth noting that there is a definite gap in the literature relating to other clinical observations.

Measurement of temperature

The oral site is most commonly used for temperature measurements in adults, but rectal and axillary temperatures are also recorded when the oral route is not possible. The body temperature varies according to the site of measurement and it is generally accepted that axillary temperature is lower than oral, which in turn is lower than rectal temperature. Nichols *et al.* (1966) looked at the relationship of body temperature and found that there were no reliable differences between the three sites: individual variations were too pronounced to enable a fixed relationship between the sites to be established. Even when considering just one site, there can be considerable vari-

97

ations in temperature according to the exact position of the thermometer; for example Erickson (1980) found that the temperature in the area under the front of the tongue was up to 0.22°C (0.4°F) lower than in the posterior sublingual pockets (the recommended site). Closs (1987) reviews in detail the technique for oral temperature measurement.

There has been much debate about the length of time that glass thermometers need to be left in situ for the maximum temperature to register. Most nursing texts recommend insertion times of 3–5 minutes. Nichols and Kucha (1972) found that the time varied according to the age, sex, site used, febrile status of the patient and the ambient temperature. They also demonstrated that only 13% of their subjects reached a maximum recording after 3 minutes and recommend, for example, an insertation time of 8 minutes for oral temperature measurement for adult males in a room temperature of 18–24°C (65–75°F).

However, the findings of other researchers have not supported the work of Nichols and colleagues. Baker *et al.* (1984) thought that insertion times of 8 minutes were unrealistic and difficult to implement. In their work they found that there were indeed differences with longer insertion times, but that the differences (of the order of 0.1°C) were not clinically significant, in other words, it does not matter in most instances if the temperature recorded is 0.1°C lower than the patient's maximum temperature. Pugh Davies *et al.* (1986) found an insertion time of 3 minutes satisfactory for oral temperature taking.

Other factors influence the accuracy of temperature measurements. For instance, using a different thermometer each time can given false variations in temperature readings. Sims-Williams (1976) describes false variations of up to 0.3°C following the use of several different thermometers in one day. Abbey *et al.* (1978) found that thermometers varied in the length of time that they retained their accuracy. Providing thermometers conforming to British Standards are used, these problems should be minimised, as all thermometers with the BSI kite mark have an accuracy of ±0.1°C. Errors can also arise if the patient has had a hot or cold drink prior to temperature measurement, or is breathing through the mouth (Durham *et al.* 1986), and oral temperature is unreliable if the person is in a cold ambient environment.

Although the mercury in glass thermometer is the most commonly used instrument for measuring body temperature, electronic and chemical thermometers are available too. There have been many studies comparing the advantages and disadvantages of glass and electronic thermometers. The findings are sometimes contradictory; some suggest that use of electronic thermometers may be most cost effective in time and money as they can register temperatures more quickly, are more accurate and reduce the risk of cross-infection (Moorat 1976; Stronge & Newton 1980; Baker *et al.* 1984; Erickson 1980). Glass thermometers do take longer to register the maximum body temperature, but Takacs and Valenti (1982) showed that nurses use *all* the time available constructively, e.g. by taking pulse and blood pressure.

A thorough study by Pugh Davies *et al.* (1986) found no significant differences in the average accuracy of electronic and glass thermometers; they also found that there was a greater fluctuation of readings when using electronic thermometers – an important negative aspect to the use of these thermometers.

An example of a study (Closs *et al.* 1986) looking at the relevance of temperature taking to patient care in the postoperative period is discussed below.

TITLE OF ARTICLE: *Factors Affecting Perioperative Body Temperature*

Main research questions What factors influence fall in body temperature during surgery? Which patients are most at risk of developing a low body temperature? Do nurses on the ward monitor the patient's body temperature postoperatively?

Research design and method The study consisted of monitoring the pre- and postoperative body temperatures of two groups of patients (17 undergoing a cholecystectomy and 14 repair of fractured femur). A control group of adults (n=8) were subjected to the same protocol but without having surgery. Several variables were monitored to establish the existence of a relationship with the fall in body temperature, including percentage body fat, age of subject, type and duration of surgery, and the ambient temperature in theatre. Body temperature was measured the day before surgery as a baseline, and was measured again once the patient returned to the general ward.

Main findings   All patients showed a significant fall in body temperature during surgery: $0.78\pm0.13°C$ in the cholecystectomy patients and $1.2\pm0.12°C$ in the fractured femur patients. The greatest falls in temperature occurred when the ambient temperature in theatre was low and were exhibited by the older patients. However, the greater the amount of body fat, the smaller the drop in body temperature. Many patients did not have their temperature taken by the nursing staff on return to the ward, and more than 30% of patients did not have temperatures taken by the nurses during the first 4.5 hours after surgery (seven patients had temperatures below $35°C$). The patients (n=4) who subsequently developed respiratory tract infections had temperatures which were significantly higher than the rest of the group 4.5 hours postoperatively.

Implications   Ward monitoring of postoperative temperatures should be thorough to identify postoperative hypothermia or pyrexia. As elderly and thin patients were particularly prone to becoming hypothermic, it would be advisable to monitor temperature carefully both during and after surgery: maintaining body temperature at preoperative levels during surgery might prevent compromising the cardiovascular and pulmonary functions of the more frail elderly patients during the immediate recovery period. The ambient temperature in theatre is also of importance and it may be possible to raise the temperature above $20°C$ for certain patients and surgical procedures, but this would have implications for the comfort of the theatre staff.

Measurement of blood pressure

Several studies have been undertaken to examine equipment used for measuring blood pressure. Conceicao et al. (1976) looked at the accuracy of sphygmomanometers in use in a hospital in Newcastle and found that almost half had defects. Tam (1979) compared the use of a traditional mercury sphygmomanometer with two electronic ones. He found that the electronic ones were more popular with the nursing staff, but that they cost more and were less reliable than the conventional types. Tam found that the electronic sphygmomanometers gave higher readings than the mercury ones. It is in fact to be expected that different equipment gave different values for systolic and diastolic pressures – as all non-invasive methods of measuring determine blood pressure indirectly and depend on the design of the equipment.

As with taking temperatures, the actual technique of taking the blood pressure is important if reliable values are to be obtained. Blood pressure measurement procedure is discussed in O'Brien and O'Malley (1981), Thompson (1981) and Lancour (1976). Many factors affect the blood pressure and these need to be considered when recording it, e.g. exercise, anxiety, position. Mancia *et al.* (1983) showed that both systolic and diastolic pressures increased significantly (26.2 ± 2.3 mmHg, 14.9 ± 1.6 mmHg respectively) when the doctor arrived at the bedside.

Some measurement errors are random due to a poor technique or equipment, but other errors are more systematic. Wilcox (1961) looked at systematic error or bias used by the observer taking blood pressure measurements, and found wide variations between and within observers, especially for diastolic pressures. Some of the most accurate readings were obtained by statisticians who had never taken BP measurements before, but were trained in objective and accurate recording of data.

As can be seen, many studies have looked at the merits of different equipment for making observations and the accuracy or inaccuracies of the technique. Inaccuracies can stem from the equipment itself and/or the observer using the equipment (Walker and Selmanoff 1965). The parameter being monitored may also alter under various conditions. For example, blood pressure can increase if the patient is anxious. Thus, for an observation to be of use and to be meaningful in the clinical context, standardised conditions must be used.

Use of clinical observations

Few studies have considered the appropriate use, value and relevance of observations as a part of nursing care. The study looking at perioperative temperature monitoring (Closs *et al.* 1986) discussed before is one exception. Nurses are often not selective in assessing which patients need particular observations and how often, and this can result in unnecessary use of time. Sims (1965) showed that reducing the frequency of temperature measurement to a 7 a.m., 2 p.m., 7 p.m. regime saved 3500 hours per year in a 500-bedded hospital without apparent loss of diagnostic or prognostic information. Angerami (1980) also looked at the frequency of temperature observations and the most appropriate time of day for detecting pyrexias: she found that 7–8 p.m. was the most sensitive time. Unfortunately, research findings such as these are rarely implemented.

There is little information available which relates to optimum timing and frequency of blood pressure measurements although one study compared measurements taken at the beginning and end of the admission procedure (Walker 1984); both systolic and diastolic pressures were significantly lower on the second reading than on the first. This has practical implications as often the 'on-admission' observations serve as a baseline for all subsequent measurements.

Summary

Although this review has concentrated on temperature and blood pressure observations, the findings of studies looking at other observations are in general similar. For instance, Hilton (1982) looked at nurses' performances and interpretation of urine testing and blood glucose monitoring, and found that registered nurses did not perform these simple tests accurately. Accurate observations are essential in monitoring a patient's physical condition, but as seen here, studies have shown that measurement of observations is often inaccurate and inappropriately timed. Inaccuracies arise from incorrect measurement procedures, use of different equipment that is often poorly maintained, and errors on the part of the observer. Inappropriate use of observations stems from traditional routines in nursing and lack of understanding and knowledge of the significance and importance of observations, so that sometimes they are recorded when not necessary and omitted when important.

There is still a considerable need for research in this field. The emphasis of future research should lie in investigating the appropriateness and use of observations rather than in the techniques per se. Other important issues which should be explored include investigating what nurses actually 'do' with the information once they have made the observations, examining the extent to which nurses understand the importance of changes, and exploring nurses' knowledge of the clinical significance of changes in vital signs.

References

Abbey J.C. *et al.* (1978) How long is that thermometer accurate? *American Journal of Nursing*, **78**, 8, 1375–1378

Angerami E. (1980) Epidemiological study of a body temperature in patients in a teaching hospital. *International Journal of Nursing Studies*, **17**, 91–99

Baker N. *et al.* (1984) The effect of type of thermometer and length of time inserted on oral temperature measurements of afebrile subjects. *Nursing Research*, **33**, 2, 109–111

Closs J. (1987) Oral temperature measurement. *Nursing Times*, **7**, 36–39

Closs S.J., Macdonald I.A. & Hawthorn P.J. (1986) Factors affecting perioperative body temperature. *Journal of Advanced Nursing*, **11**, 739–744

Conceicao S., Ward M.K. & Kerr D.N.S. (1976) Defects in sphygmomanometers: An important source of error in blood pressure recording. *British Medical Journal*, **1**, 886–888

Durham M.L., Swanson B. & Paulford N. (1986) Effect of tachypnoea on oral temperature estimation: A replication. *Nursing Research*, **35**, 4, 211–214

Erickson R. (1980) Oral temperature differences in relation to thermometer and technique. *Nursing Research*, **29**, 3, 157–164

Hilton B.A. (1982) Nurses' performance and interpretation of urine testing and capillary blood glucose monitoring measures. *Journal of Advanced Nursing*, **7**, 509–521

Lancour J. (1976) How to avoid pitfalls in measuring blood pressure. *American Journal of Nursing*, **76**, 5, 773–775

Mancia G. *et al.* (1983) Effects of blood pressure measurements – by the doctor on patient's blood pressure and heart rate. *Lancet*, **2**, 695–698

Moorat D.S. (1976) The cost of taking temperatures. *Nursing Times*, **72**, 767–770

Nichols G.A. & Kucha D.H. (1972) Oral measurements. *American Journal of Nursing*, **72**, 6, 1091–1092

Nichols G.A., Ruskin M.M., Glor B.A. *et al.* (1966) Oral, axillary and rectal temperature determinations and relationships. *Nursing Research*, **15**, 307–310

O'Brien E. & O'Malley K. (1981) *Essentials of Blood Pressure Measurement*. Edinburgh: Churchill Livingstone

Pugh Davies S., Kassab J.Y., Thrush A.J. & Smith P.H.S. (1986) A comparison of mercury and digital clinical thermometers. *Journal of Advanced Nursing*, **11**, 535–543

Sims R.S. (1965) Temperature taking in a teaching hospital. *Lancet*, **ii**, 535–536

Sims-Williams A.J. (1976) Temperature taking with glass thermometers: a review. *Journal of Advanced Nursing*, **1**, 481–493

Stronge J.L. & Newton G. (1980) Electronic thermometers – a costly rise in efficiency. *Nursing Mirror*, **151**, 29

Takacs K.M. & Valenti W.M. (1982) Temperature measurement in a clinical setting. *Nursing Research*, **31**, 6, 368–370

Tam G. (1979) A comparison of two electronic sphygmomanometers with the traditional mercury type. *Nursing Times*, **75**, 880–885

Thompson D.R. (1981) Recording patients blood pressure: a review. *Journal of Advanced Nursing*, **6**, 283–290

Walker M. (1984) Observation in the newly admitted patient. *Nursing Times*, **80**, 29–32

Walker V.H. & Selmanoff E.D. (1965) A note on the accuracy of temperature, pulse and respiration procedure. *Nursing Research*, **14**, 1, 72–76

Wilcox J. (1961) Observer factors in the measurement of blood pressure. *Nursing Research*, **10**, 1, 4–17

Chapter 10

Pressure Area Care

PETER LOWTHIAN

The sudden emergence of a deep penetrating ulcer, with no overt event to account for it, has for centuries been a conceptual problem for bedside nurses. Superficial sores, however, can be caused by abrasive (kinetic) friction, so that they are somewhat easier to comprehend and prevent.

The 'deep' pressure ulcer as described by Groth (1942) is a particular hazard for severely debilitated and paralysed patients. Elderly patients constitute the largest group of patients at risk of these pressure sores (Jordan & Barbenel 1983), but spinally injured persons and victims of Hansen's disease are also greatly at risk. Both Arnott (1833) and Paget (1873) recognised the role of sustained pressure in causing serious 'bedsores', and the normal ways that we avoid developing these sores, by spontaneous and other subconscious movements (Exton-Smith & Sherwin 1961) help to explain why they do not often occur in persons who are relatively healthy.

Reichel (1958) explained how susceptible patients, such as paraplegics, could develop serious sacral sores when prolonged semirecumbent positions induced 'shearing' strains of the tissues over the sacrum. The tensile strains produced by shearing were also found to occur when direct pressure is applied to soft tissues (Lowthian 1970), and the stretched microvessels which result seem to explain the multiple microthrombi which are found in regions of maximum tissue distortion (Dinsdale 1973; Barton 1977). The deep ischaemic plaques produced by these microthrombi appear to account for the first stage in the development of Groth's 'deep' pressure ulcers. Other factors which appear to contribute to pressure sore development include infections, drugs and incontinence.

Many special beds and patient support systems have been developed since the nineteenth century (Bliss 1964; Lowthian 1977), but practical problems such as poor maintenance and high capital cost have caused many of these to fall into disuse. Nevertheless, when pressure sores have actually developed, it is necessary strictly to limit pressure distortion on the sore, and a sophisticated patient support system is indicated (Rogers 1978).

It has been estimated that approximately 6–10% of all patients have pressure sores at any one time (Jordan & Barbenel 1983). In order to check the prevalence figures, but principally to discover how pressure sores are managed, David (1984) conducted a large-scale survey in which data were collected, by observation and by a 'five-minute' questionnaire, from randomly selected hospital units in four UK regional health authorities. A total of 132 hospitals and 737 wards were visited. Sores were defined by grade (1 to 4), the system of grading being based on that used by Lowthian (1979). The nurse in charge of care on each ward was asked questions about the patients with sores. These included the reported position and grade of the sore, or sores, the duration of the sores, the prescribed treatment, and the person who prescribed the treatment.

The overall prevalence of sores was 6.6%; in geriatric wards the prevalence was 9%. The majority of the sores were of grades 2 and 3, and less than 5 cm in diameter. A total of 1506 sores were reported, on 885 patients, and the majority were either over pelvic prominences (58%) or on the heels (22%). The responsibility for prescribing treatment for the sores was found to be largely left with nurses (82% of the 1506 sores).

Eighteen different cleansing agents were used for cleaning sores, the most commonly applied being soap and water (36%), saline (26%) and Savlon (14%). Ninety-eight different preparations were employed for being left in contact with the sores. The most frequently used of these were povidone iodine, proflavine and magenta paint. Desloughing agents were also in use, the most popular being eusol-containing preparations, followed by Aserbine and Debrisan. Only 51% of the sores were covered by a dressing, and this was usually either a dry gauze dressing or 'non-stick' gauze.

The variety of preparations and cleansing agents used on pressure sores suggests that the principles of optimum wound healing are poorly understood by most of the people involved in treating the pressure sores, and the survey has shown that this is largely nursing staff. The practice of leaving sores uncovered and washing them with soap and water should be discouraged. Not only may this practice allow cross-infection with resistant bacteria, but the drying effect of exposure will generally delay the process of healing (Torrance 1986) and exacerbate the sore by allowing it to adhere to bedding materials.

Objective assessment of the most promising preparations and dressings requires controlled trials similar to the careful work by Taylor *et al.* (1974), who showed that a twice-daily 500-mg dose of oral vitamin C was more effective than a control placebo for healing pressure sores. In this study, sore sizes were measured by photograph in order to provide objective evidence of improvement.

Usually about 25% of patients develop sores soon after hospitalisation in geriatric admission units (Bliss *et al.* 1966), and great efforts are needed to reduce this incidence. Hibbs (1982) has shown the value of a weekly register of pressure sores in heightening nursing and medical staff's awareness of the problem, and reducing the incidence of new sores. This confirms the work of Eusanio (1976). A more recent campaign by Isles (1986) has provided further confirmation of the value of monitoring sores and motivating nurses to prevent them. Isles made use of the Norton Scale (Norton *et al.* 1975), although the original scale has, over the years, been criticised for being too subjective and many additions and alterations to the basic scale have appeared. Aetiological research in the late 1970s suggested a new risk-assessment scale. This is known as the Pressure Sore Prediction Score, and it has been found to be especially useful for assessing the pressure sore risk of orthopaedic patients (Lowthian 1987).

Once identified, high-risk patients should be nursed on special support systems or given regular help in changing their position, rubbing and local applications being of little or no value (Norton *et al.* 1975). Major shifts of body weight every

2 hours have proved difficult to maintain (Bliss *et al.* 1966), but where nursing resources are very scarce, even small shifts of body weight, organised in a logical sequence (Brown *et al.* 1985), may help to prevent pressure sores. An overview of research-based approaches to maintaining healthy skin can be found in Redfern (1986).

The general purpose patient support systems (beds and mattresses) on which most patients are nursed can help to cause pressure sores (Lowthian 1977). Recent attempts to improve these support systems range from the relatively expensive Air-Wave alternating pressure system (Exton-Smith *et al.* 1982) to inexpensive polyester fibre auxiliary mattresses, such as the Silicore (Daechsel & Conine 1985). A particular attempt to improve the general purpose patient support system, which was funded by the Department of Health and Social Security, is described below. This project (Scales *et al.* 1982) resulted in the production of the Vaperm mattress.

TITLE OF ARTICLE: *'Vaperm' Patient-Support System: A New General Purpose Hospital Mattress*

Main research question   How can the varied requirements of a general purpose hospital mattress, and the bed on which it is used, be successfully combined with a specific requirement to provide a compliant and comfortable support?

Research design and method   The main investigation involved the use of special 'indenters' which modelled the effect of a patient resting on a mattress. Pressures measured on the spherical surfaces of these indenters, when pressed against the mattress under test, were found to be comparable with pressures under the buttocks of volunteers resting on the mattress.

Over a period of 10 years the Vaperm mattress and its ventilated mattress base (on a 'King's Fund' bed) were developed and tested. This included a number of pilot clinical trials and resulted in the new mattresses becoming very popular with nursing staff at the Royal National Orthopaedic Hospital, Stanmore. Insufficient funding prevented a definitive clinical trial, but the indenter system was used to compare the new mattress, in a controlled environment, with the well-known DHSS specification mattress and with various other mattresses. It was also possible to check the effect of sheets and drawsheets on the mattresses. Other laboratory tests, some conducted by commercial companies cooperating in the development of the system, checked the mattress assembly for water vapour permeability, fire resistance, static electricity and durability.

Main findings   The indenter tests showed that peak pressures on the new Vaperm mattress assembly were considerably lower than those on the DHSS mattress. Under a standard load, the main indenter gave peak pressures on the DHSS mattress of about 80 mmHg, while on the new mattress the peak pressures were in the region of 40 mmHg. The Vaperm mattress, on its ventilated base, was also found to have good water vapour transmission as well as being flame retardant. Extensive clinical experience with the Vaperm mattress has supported the laboratory findings.

Implications   The relatively low cost of the Vaperm mattress assembly and its improved fatigue properties suggest that it will be feasible to use as a general purpose patient support system. These, or similar mattresses, which can be shown to reduce patient support interface pressures to acceptable levels, while satisfying the other stringent requirements of general purpose support systems, should greatly reduce the incidence and severity of pressure sores. They should also improve patient comfort. Nurses do, however, need to recognise when a mattress has fatigued so that their patients do not acquire pressure sores by 'grounding' or 'bottoming' on the rigid base of the hospital bed.

Pressure sores can nearly always be prevented if the patients at risk are identified, and regular positional changes are combined with the use of a suitable range of patient support systems. For patients with a high risk, as well as for those with existing sores, a sophisticated support such as the Mediscus (LALBS) airbed may be needed.

Summary

The care of pressure areas needs to be based on a clear understanding of predisposing factors leading up to the development of pressure sores, so that practices which are harmful are abandoned, and measures are taken to prevent sores occurring. While special beds can help avoid the harmful distortions caused by pressure and 'shearing' forces, many of them fail to satisfy the various other requirements of an efficient patient support system.

Recent studies show that the prevalence of sores in hospitalised patients is about 7%. The incidence of new sores amongst newly admitted elderly patients may be as high as 25%. Reliable measures to reduce these figures include a weekly register of sores, identification of patients most at risk, regular shifts of body weight and introducing improved general purpose patient support systems.

The treatment of established sores is an area which merits much further research. There is a need to instigate well-designed controlled trials of different substances and to measure the effects of incorporating treatment regimes based on established principles of wound healing into the regular nursing care of patients with pressure sores. When patients at risk are identified, and regular positional changes can be combined with a suitable range of patient support systems, it should be possible both to prevent and halt the development of serious pressure sores. Further research is needed to find the best cost-effective range of support systems, and the most effective nursing measures for patients at risk.

References

Arnott N. (1833) *Elements of Physics or Natural Philosophy*, Vol. 1. London: Longman, Rees, Orme, Brown and Green

Barton A.A. (1976) The pathogenesis of skin wounds due to pressure. In Kenedi R.M., Cowden J.M. and Scales J.T. (Eds) *Bed Sore Biomechanics*. London: Macmillan

Bliss M.R. (1964) A consideration of mechanical methods of preventing bedsores in elderly patients. *Gerontology Clinics*, **6**, 10–21

Bliss M.R., McLaren R. & Exton-Smith A.N. (1966) Mattresses for preventing pressure sores in geriatric patients. *Monthly Bulletin of the Ministry of Health and the Public Health Laboratory Service*, **25**, 238–268

Brown M.M., Boosinger J., Black J. & Gaspar T. (1985) Nursing innovation for prevention of decubitus ulcers in long term care facilities. *Plastic Surgical Nursing*, **5**, 2, 57–64

Daechsel D. & Conine T.A. (1985) Special mattresses: effectiveness in preventing decubitus ulcers in chronic neurologic patients. *Archives of Physical Medicine and Rehabilitation*, **66**, 246–248

David J. (1984) Clinical forum – tissue breakdown. *Nursing Mirror*, **158**, 10, Suppl.

Dinsdale S.M. (1973) Decubitus ulcers in swine: light and electron microscopy study of pathogenesis. *Archives of Physical Medicine and Rehabilitation*, **54**, 51–56

Eusanio P.L. (1976) Monitoring skin care eliminates decubitus ulcers. *American Health Care Association Journal*, **1976**, 50–51

Exton-Smith A.N. & Sherwin R.W. (1961) The prevention of pressure sores – significance of spontaneous bodily movements. *Lancet*, **ii**, 1124–1126

Exton-Smith A.N., Wedgwood J., Overstall P.W. & Wallace G. (1982) Use of the 'Air Wave System' to prevent pressure sores in hospital. *Lancet*, **i**, 1288–1290

Groth K.E. (1942) Klinishe beobachtungen und experimentelle studien uber die Entstehung des Dekubitus. *Acta Chirurgica Scandinavica*, **76**, 126–200

Hibbs P. (1982) Pressure sores: a system of prevention. *Nursing Mirror*, **155**, 5, 25–29

Isles J. (1986) An eradication campaign. *Nursing Times*, **82**, 32, 59–62

Jordan M.M. & Barbenel J.C. (1983) Pressure sore prevalence. In Barbenel J.C., Forbes C.D. and Lowe G.D.O. (Eds) *Pressure Sores*. London: Macmillan

Lowthian P.T. (1970) Bedsores – the missing links? *Nursing Times*, **66**, 46, 1454–1458

Lowthian P.T. (1977) A review of pressure sore prophylaxis. *Nursing Mirror*, **144**, 11 (Suppl.), vii–xv

Lowthian P.T. (1979) Pressure sore prevalence. *Nursing Times*, **75**, 358–360

Lowthian P.T. (1987) The practical assessment of pressure sore risk. *Care, Science and Practice*, **5**, 4, 3–7

Norton D., McLaren R. & Exton-Smith A.N. (1975, reprint) *An Investigation of Geriatric Nursing Problems in Hospital*. Edinburgh: Churchill Livingstone

Paget J. (1873) Clinical lecture on bed-sores. *The Students' Journal and Hospital Gazette*, 1873, 144–146

Redfern S. (1986) Maintaining healthy skin. In Redfern S. (Ed.) *Nursing Elderly People*. Edinburgh: Churchill Livingstone

Reichel S. (1958) Shearing force as a factor in decubitus ulcers in paraplegics. *J. Amer. Med. Assoc.*, **166**, 762

Rogers E.C. (1978) Nursing management in relation to beds used within the national spinal injuries centre for the prevention of pressure sores. *Paraplegia*, **16**, 147–153

Scales J.T., Lowthian P.T., Poole A.G. & Ludman W.R. (1982) 'Vaperm' patient-support system: A new general purpose hospital mattress. *Lancet*, **ii**, 1150–1152

Taylor T.V., Rimmer S., Day B., Butcher J. & Dymock I.W. (1974) Ascorbic acid supplementation in the treatment of pressure-sores. *Lancet*, **ii**, 544–546

Torrance C. (1986) The physiology of wound healing. *Nursing*, 3rd series, **3**, 5, 162–168

Chapter 11

Nurse–Patient Interaction

JILL MACLEOD CLARK

The contact, interaction and communication that take place between nurses and their patients and clients form the heart of nursing practice. It is perhaps because nurse–patient interaction is so central to our understanding of nursing that it has been the subject of a wide variety of recent research studies.

Much of the early interest in nurse–patient communication was generated as a result of the numerous patient satisfaction surveys which were undertaken in the 1960s and 1970s. A consistent finding of these studies was that patients were more critical about poor communication than about any other aspect of their care in hospital (Cartwright 1964; Raphael 1969; Skeet 1970).

Many of the early studies of nursing workload (Rhys-Hearn & Potts 1978) addressed the issue of nurse–patient interaction through activity analyses but the data produced were purely quantitative, that is, they measured the amount of time being spent by nurses on different tasks or activities and said nothing about the quality of the interaction. Since communication is so central to nursing, it seems likely that the quality of nurse–patient interaction will be related to the quality of care a patient receives. More recent research in the area of nurse–patient interaction has tended to focus, therefore, on the quality of the interaction as well as on the quantity.

All studies of nurse–patient interaction inevitably use some form of observation as a method of collecting the necessary data. Observation techniques vary widely. Observers may watch one or more individuals and record the interactions using field notes or structured observation schedules. Increasingly, material for this kind of research is collected using sophisticated audio or video-tape equipment and then subjected to a leisurely post-hoc analysis. Other researchers have adopted the role of participant observer and collected data in the form of comprehensive field notes. Many use a combination of approaches and supplement their observation data with information from interviews and questionnaires. All these approaches have something to offer in terms of broadening our knowledge base and understanding of the complex processes of nurse–patient interaction. In this chapter an overview is given of a selection of studies employing a range of data-collection methods in a variety of care settings.

Interaction in the community

Until recently there has been little research which has concentrated on communication between nurses and their clients in the community. However, the emphasis in nursing is becoming more orientated towards community care and this is now an area which is receiving more attention. Work by McIntosh (1981), using observation schedules, and Kratz (1978) described the dominance of task-related conversations between district nurses and their clients. Both studies also documented the stereotyped and clichéd nature of these interactions. These findings were confirmed by Jerrett (1978) when observing the care given to children and their parents in a home care scheme.

   Montgomery-Robinson (1986) used audio-tape recordings and detailed sociological analysis of 28 conversations which took place between health visitors and clients. This study raises some important questions about possible mismatch between the idea of the health visitor as a 'family visitor' and the reality of health visiting practice.

Interaction with the elderly

An increasing proportion of patients in hospital is aged 75 years or over. It is important, therefore, that all nurses are aware of the way in which they communicate with the elderly. Early studies in this area make depressing reading, with researchers finding a consistent picture of minimal social interaction between nurses and their elderly patients (Norton et al. 1962; Adams & McIlwraith 1963). In a more recent study, Wells

(1980) found that an average 4% of the nurses' time was spent in personal contact with the patient. Personal contact was defined as any instance where nurses and patients were interacting socially in the absence of any other specific nursing activity. The findings from the analysis of tape-recorded conversations between nurses and geriatric patients echoed those of the earlier studies. She found that 50% of the exchanges lasted for less than 25 seconds and the average duration of the remainder was just under 1½ minutes. Three-quarters of all the verbal interaction occurred when nurses were giving physical care.

In a participant observation study of geriatric nursing, Baker (1978) found that nurses employed a 'routine' style of interaction with their patients which perpetuated the limited communication pattern seen. Fairhurst (1978) described a similar phenomenon of routinised and ritualised verbal interaction between nurses and elderly patients in another participant observation study.

Researchers have also focused attention on the importance of non-verbal communication and touch in the care of the elderly. Le May and Redfern (1987) observed and analysed the amount of touch that occurred between nurses and elderly patients using a complex structured observation instrument. They found that most of the physical contact was instrumental or task-related rather than taking place in its own right as an expressive or therapeutic activity.

Many of the developments in geriatric care, such as reality orientation and rehabilitation programmes, will only succeed in the context of skilled and adequate communication. With the increasing numbers of elderly in the population, it is clearly vital that the issues of improving communication between nurses and elderly patients are addressed.

Interaction with psychiatric patients

Much of the early work on the observation of nurse–patient interaction was carried out in the context of psychiatric care. Altschul (1972) undertook a sociometric analysis of interactions, looking for a link between frequency and duration of contact with the formation of relationships. Altschul found that patients suffering from organic mental disorders, that is, those whose mental disorder was combined with physical illness, received more contact with nurses than depressed or neurotic patients. The amount of time that nurses spent in interaction with patients decreased with seniority. It was also found that a few patients monopolised communication time while some appeared never to interact with the nurses. Cormack (1976) reported similar findings, with one-third of the patients he observed monopolising over three-quarters of the total interaction time. Cormack also found that, on average, charge nurses spent just 13% of their total working time in one-to-one communication with patients. He also found that certain groups of patients, the depressed, neurotic and paranoid, received less contact with nurses than did other patients.

These findings were reinforced and illuminated in a study by MacIlwaine (1983), who undertook a research project to examine the role of the nurse in relation to the neurotic patient. In this study, 24 patients were asked to wear a radio-microphone and then interactions with nurses were tape-recorded. Communication with nurses was typified by brevity and the fact that it tended to occur around specific times and events such as mealtimes and drug rounds. There was little or no evidence of nurses undertaking a therapeutic function with these patients. MacIlwaine suggests that the findings of this research illustrate the need for nurses to be helped to develop the skills required to fulfil a therapeutic communication role.

Interaction in general hospital settings

One or two observation studies have been carried out in each of a wide variety of general hospital settings. Once again the findings appear remarkably consistent, in spite of differences in research approach and nursing context. Stockwell (1972) observed the interaction between nurses and patients whilst investigating the concept of 'popular' and 'unpopular' patients and she found that communication was task-related and superficial. In a later study, Faulkner (1979) explored nurse–patient verbal interaction in a much more detailed way. Data were collected from general medical wards using a sophisticated tape-recorder, and conversations were coded post hoc according to whether they were task-orientated, social or disease orientated. The average length of interaction was between 2 and 3 minutes and conversations with male patients were shorter than those with female patients. Faulkner found that nurses tended to avoid answering patients' questions or queries and that this 'avoidance' was generalised regardless of the sensitivity or threat of the topic of the conversation.

In a study using similar methodology, Macleod Clark (1983) undertook an in-depth investigation of nurse–patient verbal interaction on surgical wards.

TITLE OF ARTICLE: *Nurse–Patient Communication: An Analysis of Conversations from Surgical Wards*

Main research questions What is the content of one-to-one (dyadic) nurse–patient verbal interactions on surgical wards? What are the dynamics of these conversations and what verbal strategies are employed by nurses?

Research design and method Data were collected from surgical wards in three hospitals in the form of audio-tape and video-tape recordings and observation schedules and field notes. Trained and untrained nursing staff were included and recordings were made of one nurse at a time during 2-hour periods. All activities were observed and recorded on an observation schedule and all contact that the nurse had with any patient during that time was recorded. A sample of 56 hours, out of a total of 180 recorded hours from the audio-tape data base, was extracted to represent a complete 14-hour working day for both student nurses and staff nurses on male and female wards. These data were then subjected to a systematic quantitative and qualitative analysis process in order to detect patterns and structure and to gain insight into the dynamics of the verbal interaction.

Main findings The average length of each student nurse–patient interaction was 2.01 minutes, with conversations between trained nurses and patients lasting an average of 1.36 minutes. During each 2-hour session, student nurses spent an average of 21.72 minutes in verbal interaction with patients, while trained nurses spent an average of 15.52 minutes. Over 80% of all interactions were initiated by the nurses and 72% were associated with the occurrence of nursing tasks. The topic of nearly three-quarters of all conversations centred around some aspect of treatment of care. Only 1.3% were related to emotional or psychosocial matters.

A qualitative analysis of the data was undertaken using a

framework of encouraging and discouraging verbal strategies. Overall, the nurses' interaction with patients tended to discourage communication. Questions to patients were overwhelmingly closed or leading and nurses were found to use few strategies which reinforced patients in conversations.

Implications The findings from this research indicate that, on the wards studied, nurse–patient interaction was limited in terms of both quantity and quality. Moreover, nurses displayed little evidence of skills which encourage communication, while demonstrating the frequent use of strategies which block or discourage further communication. These findings reinforce those of earlier, more general studies which have identified restricted patterns of nurse–patient interaction. They have also provided a starting point for developing an understanding of the processes involved, issues such as control and avoidance and the need for increasing the amount of time allocated to the teaching and assessment of communication skills in nurse education programmes.

The themes of avoidance and control have often been identified in studies of interaction between nurses and patients with cancer, many of whom are cared for in general ward settings. In their seminal study, Glaser and Strauss (1964) observed that nurses were reticent in their communications with dying patients. Bond (1983) observed nurses' conversations with patients on a radiotherapy ward and found that female patients received twice as many and longer interactions than male patients. Patients who required a large amount of physical care had most contact with nurses, although the length and content of these interactions were similar to those with all patients, in that they were limited in content and duration. Bond observed nurses using a variety of evasive tactics when dealing with difficult or sensitive issues.

Similar patterns of interaction were also described by Ashworth (1980) in her investigation of communication between nurses and patients in five intensive care units. This study is one of the few which have addressed non-verbal as well as verbal communication, but once again the findings demonstrated that nearly all communication between nurses and patients tended to be limited and superficial.

Summary

There is no doubt that, in the future, changes in our society and changing attitudes towards health care issues will place more emphasis on the nurse's ability to communicate effectively. Nurse–patient interaction will assume ever greater importance in the context of developing a health education/promotion role for all nurses and in helping patients and clients take responsibility for their own health care.

The studies overviewed in this chapter are remarkable for the consistency of their findings. Regardless of type of nurse and context of nursing care, nurse–patient interaction has been found to have many limitations. There is also similar evidence from areas not covered here, such as mental handicap nursing (see Chapter 5).

To date, nearly all studies of nurse–patient interaction have been descriptive. Over time, the methods of data collection and levels of analysis have become increasingly sophisticated and some truly qualitative analyses have been attempted. We now have an accumulated body of knowledge at a descriptive level and the time has now come to turn our attention in new directions. The next challenge is to address the issue of whether a relationship exists between the content and quality of an interaction and the outcome of that interaction in terms of patient or client well-being. Some preliminary work on this question is currently being undertaken on the link between the content of nurses' health education interventions and outcomes such as changes in patients' or clients' smoking behaviour (Macleod Clark et al. 1987).

Much more emphasis also needs to be placed on the role and function of non-verbal communication in nursing care. There is some evidence to suggest that the use of massage by nurses can result in significant pain relief in cancer patients, and this is an area of communication research which merits further investigation.

Last but not least, the most effective ways of improving nurse–patient interaction through different approaches to communication skills training should be explored. The findings from such research could influence the quality of nursing care for future generations.

References

Adams G.F. & McIlwraith P.L. (1963) *Geriatric Nursing*. Oxford: Oxford University Press

Altschul A. (1972) *Patient–Nurse Interaction*. Edinburgh: Churchill Livingstone

Ashworth P. (1980) *Care to Communicate*. London: Royal College of Nursing

Baker D. (1978) Attitudes of nurses to the care of the elderly. Unpublished PhD thesis, University of Manchester

Bond S. (1983) Nurses' communication with cancer patients In: Wilson Barnett J. (Ed.) *Nursing Research, Ten Studies in Patient Care*. Chichester: John Wiley & Sons

Cartwright A. (1964) *Human Relations and Hospital Care*. London: Routledge and Kegan Paul

Cormack D. (1976) *Psychiatric Nursing Observed*. London: Royal College of Nursing

Fairhurst E. (1978) *Talk and the Elderly in Institutions*. Paper presented to the Annual Conference of Social and Behavioural Gerontology, September 14–16 1978, Edinburgh

Faulkner A. (1979) Monitoring nurse–patient conversation on a ward. *Nursing Times*, Occasional Papers, **75**, 23, 95–96

Glaser B.G. & Strauss A.L. (1964) Awareness contexts and social interaction. *American Sociological Review*, **29**, 679–699

Jerrett M. (1978) Report of research activities. Unpublished report. University of Edinburgh, Nursing Studies Department

Kratz C.R. (1978) *Care of the Long Term Sick in the Community*. Edinburgh: Churchill Livingstone

Le May A.G. & Redfern S.J. (1987) A study of non-verbal communication between nurses and elderly patients. In Fielding P. (Ed.) *Research in the Nursing Care of Elderly People*. Chichester: John Wiley & Sons

MacIlwaine H. (1983) Communication patterns of female neurotic patients. In Wilson Barnett J. (Ed.) *Nursing Research, Ten Studies in Patient Care*. Chichester: John Wiley & Sons

McIntosh J. (1981) Communicating with patients in their own homes. In Macleod Clark J. and Bridge W. (Eds) *Communication in Nursing Care*. Chichester: John Wiley & Sons

Macleod Clark J. (1983) An analysis of nurse–patient conversations on surgical wards. In Wilson Barnett J.C. (Ed.) *Nursing Research, Ten Studies in Patient Care*. Chichester: John Wiley & Sons

Macleod Clark J., Kendall S. & Haverty S. (1987) Helping nurses develop their health education role. *Nurse Education Today*, **7**, 63–68

Montgomery-Robinson K. (1986) Accounts of health visiting. In White

A. (Ed.) *Research in Preventive Community Care*. Chichester: John Wiley & Sons

Norton D., McLaren R. & Exton-Smith A.N. (1975, reprint) *An Investigation of Geriatric Nursing Problems in Hospital*. Edinburgh: Churchill Livingstone

Raphael W. (1969) *Patients and their Hospitals*. London: King Edward's Hospital Fund for London

Rhys-Hearn C. & Potts D. (1978) The effects of patients' individual characteristics upon activity times for items of nursing care. *International Journal of Nursing Studies*, **15**, 23–50

Skeet M. (1970) *Home from Hospital*. London: Dan Mason Nursing Research Committee

Stockwell F. (1972) *The Unpopular Patient*. London: Royal College of Nurses

Wells T.J. (1980) *Problems in Geriatric Nursing Care*. Edinburgh: Churchill Livingstone

Chapter 12

Patient Teaching

JENIFER WILSON-BARNETT

In the first volume of *Research for Nursing*, references to patient teaching and information-giving studies were to be found under the broad heading of communication research. The rate of development and progress in this area during the past few years has been such that we have chosen to single out patient teaching as a discrete topic for discussion. The reason for this is that patient teaching represents one of the few aspects of nursing which have been subjected to rigorous analysis through original and replicated research. We thus have within this topic a developed body of knowledge.

Patient teaching can be defined as the process of increasing patients', or clients', understanding about their state of health, disease, treatment and rehabilitation by giving specific information in a planned and structured way. Recently, there has been an impressive growth in the volume of research which has attempted to evaluate the effect of teaching on a patient's or client's well-being.

Many of the studies in this area have employed a quasi-experimental design involving patients with similar conditions who are randomly allocated to either experimental or control groups. The experimental group members then receive the patient teaching input while the control group members receive routine treatment. All the patients are then compared in terms of variables such as their knowledge and understanding of their condition and treatment, self-care behaviour, motivation, and physiological or psychological measures of well-being.

One major area of research is that of the preparation of patients through teaching before surgery or stressful diagnostic procedures. The rationale of these studies is that the promotion of knowledge/understanding will reduce stress and enhance recovery. Classic studies in this category include those by Hayward (1975) and Wilson-Barnett (1978), and reviews of the area can be found in CURN (1980), Mathews and Ridgeway (1981) and Wilson-Barnett (1984).

Over time, studies have evolved in both scope and sophistication, but most importantly in their relevance to individual patient's needs. For instance, when reviewing experimental studies explicitly designed to evaluate teaching, Wilson-Barnett (1983) found that earlier work focused on simply giving more knowledge to patients, with the assumption that this increased knowledge per se might increase their feelings of confidence or participation. Knowledge did increase, but other effects were rarely demonstrated. Later work has tended to become more ambitious by aiming to meet the learning needs of individuals and also sometimes their relatives, in a way which could more profoundly affect coping and recovery.

Various types of information and instruction have been tested for their effects. It seems that those interventions which involve the patient in preparatory rehearsal or physical exercise are more helpful than those which simply explain what will happen. Beyond this, Johnson's (1983) review of her work demonstrates that providing an account of the patient's imminent experiences, such as the sensations, prior to the event helps to reduce stress and hasten recovery in most situations. Tailoring the material to the individual needs of the patient is also essential. For example, Ridgeway and Mathews (1983) found that when patients' own specific worries were explored in discussion and appropriate guidance on coping was provided, benefits to patients were increased: they appeared to be less worried, experienced less pain and their recovery was hastened. Important lessons for patient teaching in general can be learned from this area of research. Subject matter must be relevant to the needs of individual patients, spoken and written information is useful, and, if the teaching is provided in group sessions, then individual patients will benefit from the opportunity to discuss their own worries and coping strategies.

Some research has been undertaken to investigate the effectiveness of different teaching methods and approaches in increasing patients' knowledge and ability to cope. For example, it has been shown that individual teaching sessions, group seminars and discussions and lectures can all help improve patients' knowledge and self-care behaviour (Salzer 1975; Knudson *et al.* 1981). Sechrist (1979) demonstrated an increase in knowledge by using repeated teaching sessions and found that patients definitely appreciated this provision.

Booklets have also been evaluated as they have clear advantages as repeated patient and family reference material. Both Rahe *et al.* (1975) and Gregor (1981) studied patients recovering from myocardial infarction. Rahe's small-scale study did not include a comparison group, although patients reported that the booklets were valuable. Gregor's study of 100 patients showed that those who received a booklet achieved higher knowledge scores in the short and longer term.

It is probably fair to say that much of the early work on the use of booklets was motivated by members of the health care team eager to enhance patient compliance (that is, to take and act on advice and adhere to treatments). For example, an evaluation of individualised teaching programmes by Haynes *et al.* (1976) showed that compliance with medications and advice can be improved when careful instruction is given. This may seem unsurprising, but researchers obviously also need to explore other reasons for non-compliance such as side-effects, patients' deliberate judgements and their lack of faith in treatments. The research which as been undertaken in this area has consistently shown that improved compliance can be achieved by simplifying instructions and advice, working on a mutually agreed contract for changing behaviour, and including the spouse in relevant sessions (Dracup *et al.* 1984).

Helping patients and their family adjust to chronic disorders is perhaps the greatest current challenge for nurses. Patient teaching has a key role to play, and research studies which have involved the design and evaluation of packages or booklets are becoming more common. Some early studies only succeed in demonstrating an increase in knowledge, rather than skills or adjustment (Hentinen 1979), but others have succeeded in enhancing skills and controlling symptoms – Levine *et al.* (1979) with hypertensive people and Levine and Britten (1973) with haemophilia sufferers. It is not surprising that only a few studies show these more lasting and meaningful changes in association with experimental intervention. Skills may be difficult to acquire, and adjustment to chronic illness takes time and other resources. Skills are also difficult to assess, and 'adjustment' is certainly a complex outcome criterion which defies easy measurement.

One study worthy of note by a nurse (Ozbolt Goodwin 1979), although small scale, provides a few promising directions for research and practice. Twenty six patients who had undergone pulmonary surgery were included in this study, of which half were given educational booklets designed to facilitate programmed learning. Each patient could therefore cover exercises and skills according to his or her own pace and condition. Control patients received usual rehabilitation care. All these subjects suffered from long-term pulmonary dysfunction and could expect some alleviation of symptoms after surgery, yet without a regular programme of breathing and general exercises would be likely to suffer acute exacerbation of their condition. Those who used the booklet as instructed gained knowledge and skill but were also much healthier for several months after surgery, as indicated by fewer hospital visits and improved respiration function.

Using an experimental design in an applied field of research is always problematic and it can be difficult to conduct such studies using very large samples. Sample sizes in the more meaningful studies aiming to improve patients' feelings and coping (as in Ozbolt Goodwin's) are often very small. In spite of this, findings from the research have great relevance for nurses meeting the challenge of caring for individuals with chronic illness. Use of booklets as well as instruction might be criticised as differential effect cannot be measured. This approach is, however, reasonable in order to maximise the possible benefits. This also indicates that nurses rather than researchers may be able to achieve desirable effects using the same materials. Few studies involve significant others in teaching, which could well enhance the effects of teaching, as shown by Mayou *et al.* (1981), although it is recognised that researchers may find this difficult to arrange. Subsequent conversations between family members then serve to correct information and remind the patient of what has been taught.

Several of the more fundamental principles which have been derived from research over the years are reflected in the following study by Dracup and others in California (1984). This American team of nurses has worked with patients after myocardial infarction for some time. Team work in a multi-centre study with clear objectives and theoretical framework has advanced this field substantially and deserves a more detailed description here.

TITLE OF ARTICLE: *Group Counselling in Cardiac Rehabilitation: Effect on Patient Compliance*

Main research questions   What is the effect on cardiac patients of group counselling intervention based on the individual's self-concept, prescribed regime of rehabilitation, significant others' roles and a periodic review of these roles? What is the effect of increased involvement of spouses within the context of a group counselling intervention on the compliance of male cardiac patients?

Research design and methods   A three-group experimental design was employed for this study of 58 couples, one partner of each having suffered a heart attack. 17 couples were randomly assigned to counselling; for 22 couples, only the patient received counselling; and the third group of 19 couples acted as control. The group counselling sessions were based on symbolic interactionism, which 'holds that roles are constantly being formulated and redefined on the basis of interactions with others'. As the patient must alter his behaviour and role, so his wife must adopt different responsibilities. The patient must learn to adopt an 'at-risk' role by modifying his diet, exercise and living activities. Compliances are therefore dependent on accepting and adapting to role change. Group counselling was designed to facilitate this in 10 weekly sessions of 90 minutes each. Nurses acted as co-ordinators and focused the sessions on particular topics each week, such as ways of reducing anxiety, mastery of the 'risk role' and relaxation techniques.

Compliance measures included smoking, blood pressure, body weight and weekly exercise. These data were collected at baseline, after 10 weeks and at 6 months.

Main findings   'The study findings support the positive effects of a role-oriented group-counselling intervention on cardiac risk-factor compliance. Both experimental groups had significantly lower blood pressures and decreased triceps skinfold measurements at six-months follow-up' (Dracup *et al.* 1984, p. 175). However, in terms of reduction of blood pressure and body fat, patients in the second experimental group had superior results to those who met for counselling as a couple. The researchers questioned the assumption on interaction of roles and also the variation in group meetings in the different centres.

Implications This study was thoughtfully planned and executed. Researchers based their work on a thorough review of previous studies in the area and thereby achieved positive results. There are several implications for patient teaching from this study and others which have been successful. Central to this field is the interaction style of 'teaching'. No longer does a didactic lecture approach seem appropriate to individual patients' very complex needs. Expression of concern is vital in order to provide information and relevant support. Sharing this with others in groups in this cardiac study also seemed to help. Secondly, focusing on lifestyle and requisite adjustments was an obvious advance in this work. 'No man is an island', and by exploring how change for one person affects others is sensible. This 'theoretical' model enhanced the meaning and rationale for the sessions. Including the spouse was a logical step in this study but should now be considered for many others. Lastly, building from one session to another provides time and a clear sequence where adjustment may be encouraged and monitored. 'One-off' teaching should really only occur when there is absolutely no opportunity for further discussion.

Summary

In conclusion to this brief review, it is clear that work in the area of patient teaching continues to progress and is becoming more relevant to the needs of patients as well as fundamental to the work of nurses. Although much more research needs to be done, there are logical guidelines for practice emanating from these studies. Counselling skills need to be incorporated into 'teaching' sessions. No longer are the one-off lectures or information-giving sessions sufficient for most people's needs when they are trying to cope with a major life adjustment.

Now that the need for this work has been identified, and the type of intervention has been indicated, future research should focus on using practising nurses as the agents of patient teaching to demonstrate that they can be as successful as nurse researchers at facilitating patients' adjustment.

Davis (1984) attempted to train ward nurses to become proficient in preparing patients for surgery. However, the results of this 'field trial' proved difficult to evaluate, and this is an area which merits a great deal more research. There is also now much more written material available which could be used in these field trials. Certainly in the area of patient teaching, nurses have contributed well to research; we have an established body of knowledge and significant changes to practice should now follow.

References

CURN Project (1980) *Pre-Operative Sensory Preparation to Promote Recovery*. New York: Grune and Stratton

Davis B. (1984) *Pre-operative Information Giving and Patients' Postoperative Outcome: An Implementation Study*. Report for SHHD. Nursing Studies Unit, University of Edinburgh

Dracup K., Meleis A.I., Clark S., Clyburn A. & Stanley M. (1984) Group counselling in cardiac rehabilitation: effect on patient compliance. *Patient Education and Counselling*, **6**, 4, 169–177

Gregor F.M. (1981) Teaching the patient with ischaemic heart disease – a systematic approach to instructional design. *Patient Counselling and Health Education*, **3**, 2, 57–62

Haynes R.B., Gibson E.S., Hackett B.C., Johnson A.L., Sackett D.L., Taylor D.W. & Roberts R.S. (1976) Improvement of medication compliance in uncontrolled hypertension. *Lancet*, **i**, 1265–1268

Hayward J. (1975) *Information: A Prescription Against Pain*. London: Royal College of Nursing

Hentinen M. (1979) *The Development of the Self-care Ability of Diabetics: the Design Implementation and Evaluation of an Experimental Program of Instruction*, pp. 93–94. Helsinki: Saitaanhoidon Vuosikirja

Johnson J.E. (1983) Preparing patients to cope with stress while hospitalised. In Wilson-Barnett J. (Ed.) *Patient Teaching*. Edinburgh: Churchill Livingstone

Knudson K.G., Spiegel T.M. & Furst D.E. (1981) Outpatient educational programme for rheumatoid arthritic patients. *Patient Counselling and Health Education*, **3**, 2, 77–82

Levine D.M., Green L.W., Deeds S.G., Chwalow J., Russell R.P. & Finlay J. (1979) Health education for hypertensive patients. *Journal of the American Medical Association*, **241**, 1700–1703

Levine P.H. & Britten A.F.H. (1973) Supervised patient management of haemophilia. *Annals of Internal Medicine*, **78**, 195–201

Mathews A. & Ridgeway V. (1981) Personality and surgical recovery: a review. *British Journal of Clinical Psychology*, **20**, 243–260

Mayou R., MacMahon D., Sleight D. & Florence M.T. (1981) Early rehabilitation after myocardial infarction. *Lancet*, **ii**, 1399–1401

Ozbolt Goodwin J. (1979) Programmed instruction for self-care following pulmonary surgery. *International Journal of Nursing Studies*, **16**, 29–40

Rahe R.H., Scalzi C. & Shine K. (1975) A teaching evaluation questionnaire for post-myocardial infarction patients. *Heart Lung*, **4**, 759–766

Ridgeway V. & Mathews A. (1983) Psychological preparation for surgery. A comparison of methods *British Journal of Clinical Psychology*, **21**, 271–280

Salzer J.E. (1975) Classes to improve diabetic self care. *American Journal of Nursing*, **75**, 1324–1326

Sechrist K.R. (1979) The effect of repetitive teaching on patients knowledge about drugs to be taken home. *International Journal of Nursing Studies*, **16**, 51–58

Wilson-Barnett J. (1978) Patients' emotional responses to barium x-rays. *Journal of Advanced Nursing*, **3**, 37–46

Wilson-Barnett J. (Ed.) (1983) *Patient Teaching*. Edinburgh: Churchill Livingstone

Wilson-Barnett J. (1984) Alleviating stress for hospitalised patients. *International Review of Applied Psychology*, **33**, 493–503

Wilson-Barnett J. & Oborne J. (1983) Studies evaluating patient teaching: implications for practice. *Journal of Nursing Studies*, **20**, 1, 33–44

Chapter 13

Manpower Planning

JULIET HAWKES

The question 'How many nurses do we need?' has been considered important by nurse managers since the earliest days of the profession, and a national approach to an assessment of the requirements for and provision of nurses became possible with the establishment of the National Health Service. However, a co-ordinated response to this opportunity was slow in coming and the report of the Committee on Nursing (DHSS 1972) stated that:

> No reliable methods of measuring staff requirements have been developed . . . there are no generally applicable scientific criteria which can usefully be adopted by nursing and midwifery managers. They have little alternative therefore, but to bargain, often crudely, for a reasonable share of the budget and to spend their allocation in accordance with subjective judgements related to circumstances and the availability of staff at the time.

Recent interest in manpower planning has been affected by several additional factors. The predicted drop in the number of 18-year-old girls in the population, from which the majority of student nurses are traditionally drawn, may lead to acute shortages of trained nurses. The adoption of the Griffiths Report (DHSS 1983) by the NHS has disrupted the traditional nursing hierarchy and led to nursing staff often having managerial accountability to non-nurses, who are unable to rely on professional experience to inform their use of nursing staff. Finally, the emphasis within the health service on a more managerially and financially accountable approach has focused management attention on the fact that nurses are the largest group of staff, with a major co-ordinating role in patient care.

They therefore require a substantial allocation of resources. These and other factors have led to an increased emphasis on the need for information (DHSS 1983) which has focused both on the supply of nurses and the way this may be affected by population changes and proposed changes in nurse education. Information is also needed about potential demand for nurses, and the way this is affected by changes in approaches to patient care.

Research on the supply of nurses has been dominated by the concern to produce models of the flow of nurses into training, and their pattern of work once qualified. These models have been developed by the DHSS (1982) and different Regional Health Authorities (West Midlands Regional Health Authority 1979, 1980), and reveal some overlap in approach. In addition, local studies have been undertaken into various factors affecting supply, for example recruitment, wastage during and after training, sickness and absence, and the use of bank, agency and part-time staff. MacGuire's review (1969) provides a good, if dated, starting point for investigation, and Clark and Redfern (1978) and Mercer (1979) have all contributed to the debate on what constitutes a desirable level of turnover and how best to record it. Auld (1967) studied the employment of part-time nurses, and this remains the most comprehensive study on this topic to date, although interest in this area is growing in the light of an anticipated shortage of nurses. All these initiatives have been hampered by a lack of co-ordination and continuing data collection, with the result that a national picture on any of these aspects is incomplete.

Research on the demand for nurses initially started with the 'top-down' approach, and the DHSS/MAPLIN (1981), the DHSS (1982) and Regional Health Authorities (West Midlands Regional Health Authority 1979) have published guidance and advice on the methodologies available. This has involved attempts to relate manpower figures to patient activity levels and information on costing. As a result, there have been diverse developments from the use of simple ratios and norms to more complex formulae. While these are of value in strategic planning and for comparative purposes, they are often misleading and unhelpful when applied in specific local contexts. A major problem of this approach is the identification of the implications for the standard of care of a particular ratio of nurses to occupied beds.

The 'bottom-up' approach relies on estimating the demand for nursing time made by an individual patient and then aggregating this to form a total picture of the demand for nurses in a ward, department, hospital or community area. Many studies have been undertaken using this approach and a description of the earlier ones can be found in the review by Wilson-Barnett (1978). More recently, Telford has developed a system for estimating nursing manpower requirements which uses negotiated allocation of the workforce bases on nurses' subjective professional views of what staff are necessary (Telford 1979).

The Telford approach is thus very different from the traditional 'patient dependency study' in that it asks ward staff to set acceptable staffing levels for each shift in their area rather than making time counts. These estimates then form the basis of the calculation of the requirement for nurses, and have to be justified at each level of the hierarchy. The systematic rationalisation of the nurses' subjective assessments forms the basis of the method which merely makes explicit the subjective elements of all assessment of nursing workload. As it is relatively cheap and easy to carry out and incorporate a significant degree of consultation at all levels of the service, it has been welcomed as one of the more practicable approaches to estimating nursing manpower requirements (Telford 1979).

An alternative 'bottom-up' approach has been taken by some researchers, who have tried to categorise patients into groups (dependency categories) according to the average time taken to care for them. Goddard (1963) divided patients into five groups and this approach was modified by the North Eastern Regional Hospital Board (1967, 1969) to produce the Aberdeen Formula. This has since been subjected to further evaluation (Northern Regional Health Authority and South Tyneside Area Health Authority 1978). Barr produced three dependency categories based on time ratios and his work is described in Barr *et al.* (1973).

The Cheltenham study (Gloucester Area Health Authority 1982) used a system whereby each patient was categorised on a 1 to 4 scale on four different variables: mobility, hygiene, feeding and psychosocial items. A task list completed by the nurses shows which tasks they did for each patient, and how long these tasks took. Working from the relationship shown between the timings and the dependency score, the average timings were used to predict the nursing time required to nurse patients of a particular dependency. This approach allows flexibility, as the breakdown of tasks over the 24 hours can be used to predict how many nurses will be required on each shift. It can also be applied individually by each ward, so that particular characteristics or the demands of any given specialty can be accommodated. The disadvantage of this method is that it relies on collecting retrospective data within a particular ward or department and therefore reflects what has happened, rather than what should have happened. Clearly, if planning is to be orientated towards meeting future needs, it must be based on policies designed to meet *those* needs, rather than historical activity patterns.

Auld (1976) applied these methods to midwifery and concluded that their application overemphasised physical dependence, and: 'more attention should be given to assessing the provision of skills to meet psycho-social and educational needs' (p. 56). Rhys Hearn's (1977) work is more closely based on the needs of the individual, but ultimately places him or her in one of five basic care groups and one of five technical care groups. An average time is then applied to these groups and aggregated to give a ward total.

The problem with all the methods discussed so far is that none of them allows for a qualitative assessment of what the *level* of nursing should be in order to produce a particular standard of care. One researcher who has attempted to tackle this issue is Grant (1979). She undertook a study of manpower requirements which were geared to individualised patient care, and this is described below.

TITLE OF BOOK: *Time to Care: A Method of Calculating Nursing Workload based on Individualized Patient Care*

Main research question   Is it possible to introduce into a clinical area a system of calculating the daily nursing workload based on the concept of individualised patient care?

Research design and method   This study took place in Scotland on three medical wards in an acute teaching hospital. The research relied on the use of individualised nursing care plans, which were a relatively new concept in Britain at the time of the study. Care plans therefore had first to be introduced and incorporated into the ward situation before the study commenced. The ward used task allocation as the method of allocating work. The researcher divided the work of the nurses she observed into activities which were clusters of tasks, which she then timed. Once an activity had been observed and timed ten times, the mode, or alternatively the mean time, was taken as the 'suggested time' for that activity. Activities were divided into 'planned' and 'unplanned' activities according to whether they appeared in individual patients' care plans. From continuous observation of staff on the ward, it was possible to state that 73% of staff time was taken in planned activity and 27% in unplanned or general ward activity. At night the ratio of planned activity dropped to 38% but a substantial proportion of time was taken with 'general observation', reflecting the need for safe staffing levels at night in case of emergency.

Staff were asked to complete care plans for the patients and then to assess the time taken to complete the activities proposed, in the light of the suggested times previously obtained by the researcher. These times were then added up for each individual patient, then summated over all patients on the ward, and finally 30% was added to give the total nursing staff requirement.

Main findings   The study demonstrated that it was possible to measure workload through the timing of care plans, and that this method allows workload measurement to be based on what nurses should be doing rather than existing patterns of care. The method allows the requirement for nurses to be spread over the existing shift system, and it also takes account of the special role of the ward sister. The system makes allowance for a change in procedures, merely requiring the re-timing of any changed activities. Allowance can also be made for the different grades of staff involved in patient care by suggesting that the nurse responsible for drawing up the care plan notes the lowest grade of staff allowed to undertake the activity. This then allows the summation of timings in the light of the grades of staff required. Thus, skill mix is accommodated, which is becoming increasingly recognised as an important aspect of manpower planning. The system also recognises the importance of psychosocial care in relation to patients, and provided this need is identified in the care plan, allowance will automatically be made for this in the number of staff required. However, the study demonstrated that nurses found it difficult to collect the data reliably and, as a result, accurate and complete manpower information was not available over the 6 months that data were collected, which in turn reduced staff motivation towards the study. Grant concluded: 'the problems evinced in this project were due to motivation and instruction rather than lack of capability. It is thought that if the staff could see evidence of the effect of their efforts in a functioning system, such problems would be considerably lessened.' (p. 115).

The use of a computerised system was considered during this study, and would have been welcomed, as the amount of transcription and calculation involved undertaken by the researcher and the staff could then have been considerably reduced.

Implications   This was an ambitious study, in that it involved not only the introduction of a manpower information system, but also the introduction of individualised patient care planning. Experience has shown that individualised care planning is a skill with which the profession has taken some time to become totally comfortable, and even now there is a considerable variety of approach to the concept. Nevertheless, there are indications that with the growth of use of computers at ward level, and the demand for valid and reliable data on the nursing workload generated by patients in hospital and in the community, a computerised approach to care planning will become available. It is possible to envisage a system whereby nurses could compile an individualised care plan from a selection of possible goals and actions, which would have been pre-timed where possible, but which a nurse could override where she felt it appropriate to do so.

By completing the care plans of all patients on the ward, the nurse could automatically enter all the information necessary to calculate the nursing workload on that ward by grade of staff and by shift. This could then be linked to costings to assess the use a particular patient has made of health service resources during his illness, and to personnel information to give the total requirements for nursing care over time and related to staff available.

The importance of this approach to manpower planning systems lies in the appropriate interpretation of the results of using such systems. As yet there is no generally accepted way of linking the quality of nursing care that patients receive to staff numbers required. There are two fundamental problem areas: the first concerns the lack of an agreed approach to the measurement of the quality of care, as discussed in the next chapter; the second problem is the lack of a demonstrable relationship between the number of nurses present and the quality of care received.

The work of Ball *et al.* (1983) has attempted to link these elements by proposing a method of assessing patient dependency, and a method for assessing the quality of care. Both these methods could be further refined. The prospect of developing a method of assessing workload which has a feedback mechanism making it possible to demonstrate the relationship between the numbers of nurses available and the quality of care patients receive is most exciting. However, the variety of methods of calculating workload, the cumbersome data collections and the lack of an accepted national manpower planning system for nurse manpower planning illustrate the difficulties of research in this area. Nevertheless, the assessment of workload linked to requirements for nursing personnel and to outcome measures of nursing care seems the way to proceed. However, the methods to be employed to do this are dependent on further research, and it is essential that nurses are deeply involved if these methods are to reflect nursing values, and fully develop the role of the nurse.

References

Auld M. (1967) An investigation into the recruitment and integration of nursing staff in hospitals. *International Journal of Nursing Studies*, **4**, 119–169

Auld M. (1976) *How Many Nurses: A Method of Estimating the Requisite Nursing Establishment for a Hospital*. London: Royal College of Nursing

Ball J.A., Goldstone L.A. & Collier M.M. (1983) *Criteria for Care: The Manual of the North West Nurse Staffing Levels Project*. Newcastle upon Tyne: Polytechnic Products Ltd

Barr A., Moores B. & Rhys Hearn C. (1973) A review of the various methods of measuring the dependency of patients on nursing staff. *International Journal of Nursing Studies*, **10**, 195–208

Clark J. & Redfern S. (1978) Absence and wastage in nursing. Nursing Times Occasional Paper in two parts. *Nursing Times*, **74**, (11 and 12)

Department of Health and Social Security, Scottish Home and Health Department and Welsh Office (1972) *Report of the Committee on Nursing*, p. 130. Cmnd 5115. London: HMSO

Department of Health and Social Security/MAPLIN (1981) Extracts from *Wessex Strategic Planning User Manual*. Manpower Planning Department. Wessex Regional Health Authority MAPLIN Paper 81/13. London: HMSO

Department of Health and Social Security/Operational Research Service (1982) *ORS National Supply Model for Nurses: Review of the Model and Possible Areas for Further Work*. ORS/NURSD1

Department of Health and Social Security/Operational Research Service (1983) *Nurse Manpower Planning: Approaches and Techniques*. London: HMSO

Department of Health and Social Security (1983) The Griffiths Report. London: HMSO

Gloucester Area Health Authority (1982) *Total Care Dependency Study at Cheltenham General Hospital*. Unpublished Reports 1 and 2

Goddard A.A. (1963) *Work Measurement as a Basis for Calculating Nursing Establishments*. Leeds: Leeds Regional Hospital Board

Goldstone L.A., Ball J.A. & Collier M.M. (1983) *Monitor: An Index of Nursing Care in Medical and Surgical Wards*. Newcastle upon Tyne: Polytechnic Products Ltd

Grant N. (1979) *Time to Care: A Method of Calculating Nursing Workload Based on Individualised Patient Care*. London: Royal College of Nursing

MacGuire J. (1969) *Threshold to Nursing: A Review of the Literature on Nurse Training Programmes in the U.K*. Occasional Papers in Social Administration No. 30. London: Bell

Mercer G. (1979) *The Employment of Nurses. Nursing Labour Turnover in the NHS*. London: Croom Helm

North Eastern Regional Hospital Board, Scotland (1967, 1969) *Nursing Workload as a Basis for Staffing* (Scottish Health Service Studies No.3 and No.9). Edinburgh: Scottish Home and Health Department

Northern Regional Health Authority/South Tyneside Area Health Authority (1978) *Report on the Evaluation of the Aberdeen Formula for Calculating Nurse Establishments in Hospital Wards*.

Rhys-Hearn C. (1977) Nursing workload determination: Development and trials of a package. *Medical Informatics*, **2**, 2

Telford W.A. (1979) *Determining Nursing Establishments*. Health Service Manpower Review, Vol. 5, No. 4

West Midland Regional Health Authority (1979) *Using the Civil Service Manpower Planning Models on Nurse Staffing Problems*. Management Services Division Operational Research. Birmingham; West Midlands Regional Health Authority

West Midlands Regional Health Authority (1980) *Use of the Trent Nursing Formula*. MAPLIN paper 80/110. London: HMSO

Wilson Barnett J. (1978) *A Review of Patient Nurse Dependency Studies*. Nursing Research Liaison Group. London: HMSO

Chapter 14

Quality of Care

JENNIFER M. HUNT

There is a sense in which most nursing research addresses the quality of care in that nearly all such projects have the implicit and explicit aim of improving care. In this chapter, however, the concern is with specific research studies which have investigated the concept of quality as an aspect of care which is measurable in its own right and with research studies which have explored quality assurance.

The need to measure the quality of nursing care has long been emphasised. Reviews of the literature (Van Maanen 1979; Smith 1984) demonstrate that research into the quality of nursing care go back a long way, at least to the 1930s, and, indeed, as far as Florence Nightingale herself. The term 'quality assurance' represents a more recent development, and research into this area is more limited. The two topics, however, share a common literature and are closely interrelated. However, although numerous studies have been undertaken, they do not fit into any coherent pattern nor build upon each other. This is true even in the United States, where interest in the topic began earlier and has been maintained more consistently than in the United Kingdom.

There are three main reasons why research into quality lacks cohesion. Firstly, it is inherently very difficult to define 'quality of care', despite many attempts to do so. Secondly, there has been only intermittent interest in the topic, which means there is a long 'history' and considerable re-invention of the wheel. Thirdly, interest in the subject is often related to other external developments and pressures such as manpower problems, publicised incidents of poor care, legislation and cost. In the USA, this link is seen most clearly with the introduction of legislation establishing the accreditation system, and in the UK with the setting up of the Study of Nursing Care Project which specifically mentions the link with manpower problems (McFarlane 1970).

Several attempts have been made to impose some structure onto the work in this area. For example, McFarlane (1970) divided the literature on quality into three main categories. These were research studies which developed criteria of quality, theoretical work on the problem of developing criteria of quality, and general studies on the quality of nursing care. She identified 54 studies in the first category, almost all of which came from North America, and these were further subdivided into those dealing with nurse performance and those dealing with the effect of care (patient welfare).

Donabedian (1980) has made one of the most important contributions to the field of quality. Although his work has been undertaken primarily in relation to medical care, it has been adopted as a conceptual framework by the great majority of people working in this area. He identified three components of a care system – structure, process and outcome. *Structure* is defined as 'relatively stable characteristics of the providers of care, of the tools and resources they have at their disposal and of the physical and organisational settings in which they work'. *Process* is 'the set of activities that go on within and between practitioners and patients'. *Outcome* is 'a change in a patient's current and future health status that can be attributed to antecedent health care' (Donabedian 1980).

Donabedian argued that the most important component in assessing quality is process because 'the most direct route to an assessment of care is an examination of that care'. However, he does also suggest that there is a direct relationship between all three components. Bloch (1977) suggested that the process –outcome link is vital and should be seen as an entity in its own right. This emphasis on process and outcome has influenced much of the nursing research undertaken in the last 10–15 years, which has focused on the need to demonstrate cause and effect. Thus the concepts of structure, process and outcome pervade much of the literature on quality of care.

The research can also be subdivided into the following categories: identifying, defining and describing quality; measuring quality; testing/comparing different instruments; and quality assurance. These categories will be used in the following discussion of research and quality of care in nursing.

Identifying, defining and describing quality

In terms of influence, Donabedian (1980) again is perhaps the most important author, even when this influence is sometimes not acknowledged, and his more recent publications demonstrate the research basis to his work.

In the UK the RCN has taken a leading role in trying to define quality. This began in 1967 with the setting up of the Study of Nursing Care Project, with the first and last volumes of the series being attempts to define and analyse quality using both existing literature and the research studies themselves. A decade later, a working party produced two important documents: *Towards Standards* (RCN 1980) and *Standards of Care* (RCN 1981). In 1985, a further project was set up which has a group working on the development of a conceptual framework for standard setting.

Descriptive studies have been undertaken to try to identify quality through describing 'good' and 'bad' practice. An early example is Revans' (1964) work, which is important because of its attempts to look at the whole organisation. Revans' team looked at a number of different aspects – student nurse wastage, patient length of stay, attitudes and beliefs of staff – then attempted to draw these together to identify the qualities of 'good' hospitals. The studies in the Study of Nursing Care Project were designed to achieve this aim too, although with only limited success, since each researcher undertook her own study so there was no overall pattern or framework. However, each piece of work raised important issues, and questions related to quality of care and examples include Stockwell (1972), Hawthorn (1974) and Hamilton Smith (1972).

Standards of care A considerable number of the attempts to describe quality are developed in the form of standard setting. These range from broad statements such as those of the American Nurses Association (ANA) (1979a), to more specific ones such as those produced by Ayrshire and Arran Health Board (1985), detailed standards relating to a specific area of practice such as oncology nursing (ANA 1979b), care of the elderly

(City and Hackney H.A. 1987) and midwifery (Welsh Office 1985).

Although some standards may reflect or indeed be based on research, they rarely indicate where this is so. Furthermore, the impact of these standards, either in terms of the extent to which they are put into practice, or the effect of any such utilisation, has received minimal attention.

Measuring 'quality'   Studies attempting to measure quality go back a long way. An important group try to measure quality from the patients' perspective. One of the best known and earliest is Abdellah and Levine's (1957) study carried out in the USA, in which 8660 patients in 60 hospitals were surveyed using a questionnaire to find out their views on the care they received. In the UK, Raphael (1967) used in-depth unstructured interviews in the first instance to find out from patients and staff their views on nursing and other services. Overall in this study, as indeed is usually the case, 73% of patients expressed satisfaction with their care, but this overall score hides considerable variations between different groups. As a result of this initial project, a structured questionnaire was developed and used to measure satisfaction in a further study of hospital patients. The final result was the development of an attractive, simple questionnaire by the King's Fund which hospitals could use themselves.

More recently, Moores and Thompson (1986) have undertaken an extensive study of hospital patients, again with the aim of developing a useful tool for regular assessment of quality.

TITLE OF ARTICLE: *What 1357 Hospital In-patients think about Aspects of their Stay in British Acute Hospitals*

Main research questions   What do hospital patients think about their stay in hospital following discharge? In addition, can that information be obtained in such a way that quality of care can be determined and comparisons made between hospitals in order to provide a sound basis for decision taking?

Research design and method   The study was divided into seven phases, the first six of which were developmental. The purpose of this intensive work was to develop a questionnaire which was based on issues about which discharged patients were most concerned and which provided valid and reliable data on patients' perceptions of quality of care. The final questionnaire, 32 pages long, contained a wide variety of questions.

The main study was a questionnaire survey of 3456 discharged patients from seven hospitals, which varied in size from 152 to 669 beds. Patients were randomly selected from the hospital records according to an agreed sampling frame so that a representative sample was obtained in terms of specialty (orthopaedics, general medicine, general surgery), sex and time since discharge. The questionnaire was distributed through the local Community Health Council, with an accompanying note explaining that it was a joint CHC/UMIST (University of Manchester Institute of Science and Technology) project.

Main findings   There was a usable response rate of only 39%, so the findings must be treated with caution. The main finding was the wide disparity in responses between hospitals, plus in some areas a wide range of responses within an institution. In one hospital, 39% of patients said they had received no information before admission about the hospital, although on a positive note, bathroom and toilet facilities appeared in general to be satisfactory. In spite of this, in one hospital, 11% of respondents said they 'often had to queue'. General satisfaction with the nature and rapidity of nursing care was high. An interesting finding was that satisfaction levels for day and night were closely related. However, there were wide variations within institutions about the need to ask nurses for help before getting it.

Three questions focused on the relationship between patients and nurses. The response showed that good informal relationships occur when task orientation is less obvious and when the workload is lower. The majority of patients saw that, whereas medical and other support staff treated the nurses as equals, nurses treated the doctors as superiors, but medical support staff as equals.

Of most concern perhaps were the responses to questions about discharge from hospital. For example, in one hospital, 40% of respondents stated they had only a few hours warning and in the same institution 58% had to make their own arrangements. The extent of advice on leaving hospitals also appeared meagre. In the 'best' hospital only 22% said they were both told and given written instructions.

Implications of findings   The responses highlight the problems of low expectation from consumers giving rise to a high general expression of satisfaction, and a general lack of criticism of nurses and nursing even when specific aspects of nursing came under fire such as preparing the patient for going home. As a method of assessing quality, this approach clearly has limitations.

However, the ability to compare one's own hospital with others was an important part of the study. The feedback was seen as a way to stimulate necessary changes by identifying major areas of concern. Unlike many surveys, this study has resulted first in some of the hospitals concerned acting on the results and second in the questionnaire and data analysis becoming available nationwide for nurses and managers to use.

A different approach to the measurement of quality has been through the use of audit, either retrospective, concurrent or a combination of both (McFarlane 1979). The classic work on chart audit is by Phaneuf (1976) who gives an excellent account of what audit is, and what it will and will not do, and describes the process of getting a chart audit system established. Chart audit as such however is rare in the United Kingdom although used frequently as an approach in the United States and Canada. The audits most frequently found in the United Kingdom are Qualpacs and Monitor. Some use is also being made of Rush-Medicus and a number of other instruments are being developed.

Qualpacs was developed by Wandelt and Ager (1970) in the USA. It focuses on the process of care through observation of nurse–patient interaction related to a number of different dimensions of care including psychosocial, physical, general, communication and professional implication. Wainwright and Burnip (1983a, 1983b) have reported on the use of Qualpacs to measure quality before and after changes in the provision of nursing care at Burford. They observed patients and staff on two occasions in 1981 and then in 1982. The numbers in their sample were very small. The scores for each aspect ranged from 2.0 to 2.9 on the first visit and 3.8 to 4.5 on the second. Overall nurse scores also went up from 2.6 in 1981 to 4.1 in 1982, despite a reported acute staff shortage due to sickness.

Monitor was developed by Goldstone et al. (1983) as an English version of the Rush-Medicus system (Jelinek et al, 1974), which is a sophisticated and well-tested instrument developed in the USA to measure quality in acute medical and surgical units. Monitor contains 100 items relating to the structure–process–outcomes of quality, although the majority relate to process. Used appropriately, it is a valuable way of looking at quality, but it has limitations in terms of its validity and reliability. Work is now in progress to extend its use to a wider variety of settings. Several authors describe its implementation (Pullan & Chittock 1986; David & Pritchard 1987). Padilla and Grant (1982) describe a comprehensive project which utilises audit to monitor achievement of agreed protocols in terms of both process and outcome, while Carter *et al.* (1976) developed a process and outcome audit very similar to the Rush-Medicus system. Unlike Rush-Medicus, it requires no computer analysis.

Two studies of the assessment of quality which provide somewhat different approaches are by Etheridge and Packard (1976) and Majesky *et al.* (1978). Etheridge used nursing care plans to evaluate quality on an ongoing basis by recording details of care activities as they were completed. Majesky developed a tool 'patient indicators of nursing care' which equated quality with the prevention of nursing complications. In her study she recorded and gave a score to specific indicators such as infection, pressure sores etc., and measured whether such negative outcomes had increased, decreased or remained the same during the patients' stay in hospital.

Other professions have undertaken work which could be used by nurses and this includes the study by the Royal College of General Practitioners (RCGP 1985) to identify what makes a 'good' doctor, and the work undertaken at Newcastle by Hutchinson *et al.* (1985) on setting standards. However, the evaluation of audit is an area which requires a great deal more vigorous research in the future.

Studies which compare or test different instruments

A number of authors have reviewed current instruments but without determining their evaluation through research. Openshaw (1984) provides a critical review which highlights problems and compares three measures for validity and reliability, through an analysis of the measures' development. Wright (1984) and Kerr *et al.* (1985) look at models and then discuss existing methods, with particular emphasis on major instruments. Wright also includes other measures such as nursing management audit. Jacquerye (1984), as well as describing Phaneuf, Qualpacs and Rush-Medicus, gives an account of work by Horn and Swain (1976) which led to a method for evaluating the outcomes of nursing care by measuring the patients' health status. This work was based on Orem's model of nursing (1980), from which nine categories of health status dimensions were developed and normal or optimum levels of achievement were developed and described. Of the 539 items in the instrument, Jacquerye states that all are validated but only 414 have been pre-tested for reliability. Data are collected primarily through observations and interview.

Helpfully, Jacquerye also lists the advantages and disadvantages of implementing each of the methods she describes in terms of the institution's objectives and the resources required.

However, it is important to emphasise that any instrument which purports to measure quality only has value if it can be shown to be both reliable and valid. Recently, several research studies have been undertaken looking at the issues of validity and reliability. Giovannetti et al. (1986) evaluated 50 instruments and showed that only a third had supporting reliability data available. Ventura and colleagues (1980, 1982) found inter-rater reliability between Qualpacs and Rush-Medicus to be low. Correlations between the two measures indicated that the physical and psychosocial subscales were unrelated. Giovannetti and colleagues also compared three instruments, one of which was Rush-Medicus. They found that following training, inter-rater reliability was maintained when total scores were compared. However, when the subscales were analysed the findings were mixed. Correlations between the instruments were also mixed. Both authors (Ventura and Giovannetti) argue that these findings suggest that the different instruments are measuring different aspects or dimensions of quality and are derived from different conceptual frameworks. Apart from Smith (1987), who analysed three instruments prior to selecting Qualpacs for use in her study, and Barnett and Wainwright (1987), who recently discuss critically the use of Monitor, there has been little work in this area in the UK to date.

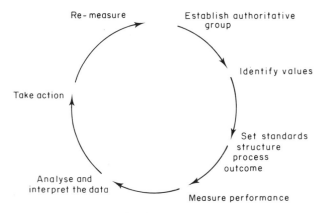

Figure 14.1 Quality assurance: the process

Quality assurance

Quality assurance is a process in which standards describing the level of quality desired and feasible are set, the level of achievement of those standards is measured, and action is taken to correct identified deficiencies. Most authors agree on the basic components of the process, although the details differ. Shaw (1986a) suggests that it consists of a cycle of activity with the three principal stages of observing practice, comparing practice with expectations, and implementing changes. More frequently it is seen as containing the steps outlined in Fig. 14.1.

Since the implementation of the Griffiths Report, quality assurance has become an important topic. Increasingly, managers and professionals are being asked to develop quality assurance programmes and to demonstrate that they are as concerned with quality as with quantity. Although the recent surge in interest makes it appear that it is a new topic, this is not so. Publications have appeared on the subject since the 1970s. The main focus has been on describing what is meant by quality assurance, how it can be achieved, and the current situation. Shaw (1986a, 1986b) has reviewed the work of the Royal Colleges, with the emphasis on medicine. A similar approach has been taken by Duncan (1985).

Articles on quality assurance and nursing are appearing more frequently, but these are not always research based. Dunne (1986) has explained clearly and simply what quality assurance means, while Kitson and Kendall (1986) link it with their research work on standards of care. Padilla and Grant (1982) have taken an interesting approach in an unusual study in which a research department tried to develop, implement and evaluate a quality assurance programme for nursing. It was based on two conceptual frameworks, Orem's theory of self-care (1980) and Kaplan and Greenfeld's (1978) criteria mapping which links patient status to nursing actions to desired outcome. They developed a model which includes identifying standards, ensuring those standards are put into practice, and then measuring whether the programme to improve nursing care had in fact done so.

There is much information available about methods of quality assurance (RCN 1987; Pearson 1987). However, overall there is little research into the effectiveness of quality assurance programmes, although Giovannetti and colleagues (1986) do suggest a model for evaluation and some research proposals are in the pipeline. It is now essential that such research is undertaken to evaluate the effectiveness of quality assurance programmes in order to determine whether the cost and effort of these initiatives are worthwhile in terms of influencing the quality of care given.

Conclusions

Although there is a vast amount of literature on standards and quality, there is very little in the way of good research. Most of the tools used to measure the quality of nursing care lack reliability and validity. Many studies are 'one-offs' and do not build on existing knowledge. Some key projects have not been followed up, possibly due to change in the political climate.

A look at the research shows that in the past it has either been undertaken by postgraduate students in order to do something about care in a particular institution or, occasionally, in response to public pressure. More recently, however, quality has become part of longer term research programmes and it is hoped that this will improve both the quality and quantity of research initiatives in this area. In addition, it has again become an important issue professionally, managerially and politically, so it is likely that more funding and resources will become available for research.

If this is to be the case, there are several areas where attention needs to be focused. First, in the light of nurses' and managers' liking for 'a measuring tool', and the current increase in such instruments, proper comparisons and evaluations of them must be carried out. This needs to be done with those tools presently in use and all new instruments should be subjected to similar rigorous scrutiny. Following on from that, research into how to introduce such tools and the impact of their use on the quality of care needs to be undertaken.

The third area to which attention needs to be paid is to the development of standards, their implementation into action and the impact on outcome. There are now many standards being developed and their value needs to be established. Fourth, research into quality assurance programmes need to be initiated, perhaps on a case study basis, again to evaluate their effectiveness.

Last, but not least, it might be better to pay less attention to seeking a global measure of nursing quality, and to focus our attention on smaller and more homogeneous parts of nursing care and getting those right. Quality is not and never can be static, so research into it needs to be flexible and fast moving. That means focusing on specific areas, then linking them together rather than trying to develop a simple quality 'score' which hides important variations.

References

Abdellah F. & Levine E. (1957) Developing a measure of patient and personal satisfaction with nursing care. *Nursing Research*, **5**, 3, 100–108

ANA (1979a) *Standards for Nursing Practice*. Kansas City: American Nurses Association

ANA (1979b) *Outcome Standards for Cancer Nursing Practice*. Oncology Nursing Society & ANA Division on Medical Surgical Nursing Practice. Kansas City: American Nurses Association

Ayrshire and Arran Health Board (1985). *Standards of Nursing Practice*. Ayrshire and Arran Health Board

Barnett D. & Wainwright P. (1987). A measure of quality. *Senior Nurse*, **6**, 3, 8–9

Bloch D. (1977) Criteria, standards, norms, clinical terms in quality assurance. *Journal of Nursing Administration*, **7**, 20–30

Carter J., Hilliard M., Castles M., Stoll L. & Cowan A. (1976) *Standards of Nursing Care: A Guide for Evaluation*. 2nd Edition. London: Springer

City and Hackney H.A. (1987) *Achievable Standards of Care for the Elderly Cared for in the Acute Assessment Wards, the Continuing Care Wards, Nursing Homes and Day Hospitals within the City and Hackney H.A.* London: City and Hackney H.A.

David J. & Pritchard P. (1987) Using Monitor. *Senior Nurse*, **6**, 4, 42–45

Donabedian A. (1980) *Explorations in Quality Assessment and Monitoring. Part 1. The Definition of Quality and Approaches to its Assessment*. Health Administration Press. Kansas City: University of Michigan

Duncan A. (1982) Quality assurance in the United Kingdom. In Selbmani H. and Uterla K. (Eds) *Quality Assessment of Medical Care*. For Robert Bosch, Stiftung Grüb H, by Bleicher Verlag

Dunne L. (1986) Defining quality assurance. *Professional Nurse*, **2**, 47–49

Etheridge P. & Packard R. (1976) An innovative approach to measurement of quality through utilisation of nursing care plans. *Journal of Nursing Administration*, **6**, 42–48

Giovannetti P. *et al.* (1986) Measuring quality of nursing care: analysis of reliability and validity of selected instruments. Unpublished report. Alberta: Faculty of Nursing, University of Alberta

Goldstone L., Ball J. & Collier M. (1983) *Monitor: an Index of the Quality of Nursing Care for Acute Medical and Surgical Wards*. Newcastle upon Tyne Polytechnic

Hamilton Smith S. (1972) *Nil by Mouth*. London: Royal College of Nursing

Hawthorn P. (1974) *Nurse, I Want my Mummy*. London: Royal College of Nursing

Horn B. & Swain M. (1976) An approach to development of criterion measures for quality health care. In American Nurses Association (Ed.) *Issues in Evaluation Research*. Kansas City: ANA

Hunt J. (1985) *Nursing Research. Does it Make a Difference*. Proceedings of Second Open Conference of WENR. London: Royal College of Nursing

Hutchinson A. *et al.* (1985) *Performance Review in Primary Care: Measuring the Effect of Standard Setting*. Unpublished report. Health Care Research Unit, University of Newcastle upon Tyne

Inman U. (1975) *Towards a Theory of Nursing Care*. London: Royal College of Nursing

Jacquerye A. (1984) Choosing an appropriate method of quality assurance. In Willis L. and Linwood M. (Eds). *Measuring the Quality of Nursing Care*. Edinburgh: Churchill Livingstone

Jelinek R., Haussman R., Hegvary S. & Newman J. (1974) *A Methodology for Monitoring Quality of Care*. Washington: Department of HEW.H.R.A. 74, 25

Kaplan S. & Greenfeld S. (1978) Criteria mapping using logic in the evaluation of processes of care. *Quality Review Bulletin*, **4**, 3–7

Kerr J., Giovannetti P. & Buchan J. (1985) Dynamics of quality assurance in nursing: a model for evaluation. In *Proceedings of Second Open Conference of the WENR*. London: Royal College of Nursing

Kitson A. & Kendall H. (1986) Quality assurance. *Nursing Times*, **82**, 29–31

McFarlane J. (1970) *The Proper Study of the Nurse*. London: Royal College of Nursing

McFarlane J. (1979) Take aim and shoot for goal. *Nursing Mirror*, **148**, Supplement, xx–xxiv

Majesky S., Bresler M. & Nishlo K. (1978) Patient indicators of nursing care. *Nursing Research*, **27**, 365–371

Moores B. & Thompson A. (1986) What 1357 hospital inpatients think about aspects of their stay in British acute hospitals. *Journal of Advanced Nursing*, **11**, 87–102

Openshaw S. (1984) Literature review: measurement of adequate care. *International Journal of Nursing Studies*, **21**, 4, 295–304

Orem D. (1980) *Nursing: Concepts of Practice*, 2nd Edn. London: McGraw Hill

Padilla G. & Grant M. (1982) Quality assurance programmes for nursing. *Journal of Advanced Nursing*, **7**, 135–145

Pearson A. (Ed.) (1987) *Nursing Quality Measurement. Quality Assurance Methods for Peer Review*. Chichester: John Wiley & Sons

Phaneuf M. (1976) *The Nursing Audit*. Connecticut: Appleton Century Crofts

Pullan B. & Chittock J. (1986) Quantifying quality. *Nursing Times*, **82**, 38–39

Raphael W. (1967) Do we know what patients think? A survey comparing the views of patients, staff and committee members. *International Journal of Nursing Studies*, **4**, 209–223

RCGP (1985) *What Sort of Doctor? Assessing Quality of Care in General Practice*. Report from General Practice No.23. London: RCGP

RCN (1980) *Standards of Nursing Care*. London: Royal College of Nursing

RCN (1981) *Towards Standards*. London: Royal College of Nursing

RCN (1987) *Nursing Quality Assurance Directory*. London: Royal College of Nursing

Revans R. (1964) *Standards for Morale: Cause and Effect in Hospitals.* Nuffield Provincial Hospitals Trust

Shaw C. (1986a) *Introducing Quality Assurance.* Kings Fund Project Paper No.64. London: King's Fund

Shaw C. (1986b) *Quality Assurance: What the Colleges are Doing.* Quality Assurance Project Report. London: Kings Fund

Smith P. (1984) Towards quality. *Senior Nurse*, **1**, 34, 10–11

Smith P. (1987) The relationship between quality of care and the ward as a learning environment. *Journal of Advanced Nursing*, **12**, 4, 413–421

Stockwell F. (1972) *The Unpopular Patient.* London: Royal College of Nursing

Van Maanen H. (1979) Perspectives and problems on quality of nursing care: an overview of contributions from North America and recent developments in Europe. *Journal of Advanced Nursing*, **4**, 377–389

Ventura M., Hageman P., Slakter M. & Fox R. (1980) Inter-rater reliabilities for two measures of nursing care quality. *Research in Nursing and Health*, **3**, 25–32

Ventura M., Hageman P., Slakter M. & Fox R. (1982) Correlations of two quality of nursing care measures. *Research in Nursing and Health*, **5**, 37–43

Wainwright P. & Burnips S. (1983a) Qualpacs at Burford. *Nursing Times*, **79**, 36–38

Wainwright P. & Burnips S. (1983b) Qualpacs the second visit. *Nursing Times*, **79**, 26–27

Wandelt M.A. & Ager J. (1970) *Quality Patient Care Scales (QUAL-PACS).* Detroit: Wayne State University

Welsh Office (1985) *Midwifery Sub-group. All Wales Nurse Manpower Planning Group. Standards of Care.* Welsh Office

Wright D. (1984) An introduction to the evaluation of nursing care: a review of the literature. *Journal of Advanced Nursing Studies*, **9**, 5, 457–467

Chapter 15

Conclusion: Research and the Future

JILL MACLEOD CLARK and LISBETH HOCKEY

From reading this volume and its earlier companion *Research for Nursing*, it must be obvious that the development of nursing research has been miraculously rapid.

The reader who has reached this final chapter will no doubt understand why we felt it necessary, in this volume, to invite a group of specialists to contribute the chapters within their own areas of work. Not only has the quantity of research increased, but the designs and methods used have become increasingly sophisticated.

In peering into the future of nursing research we are, inevitably, confronted by nursing itself. The future of nursing and the research which constitutes its body of knowledge are, or should be, inextricably linked. It is no longer possible to pretend that the one can survive, let alone thrive and develop, without the other. This chapter, therefore, concerns itself with the future of our profession, which claims to value and continues to emphasise its research base.

The previous volume concluded with a chapter on research as a change agent. We would reiterate our conviction that this potential of research to act as an agent of change must be the ultimate goal. Organisational change will happen in any case – it is inevitable. However, if we would like such change to be rooted in facts rather than be based on mere whims of the imagination, research must be encouraged.

In contrast to the rapidity and frequency of organisational change, change in clinical care patterns has continued to be slow. Convention and habitual routine rather than research-based knowledge have tended to guide practice. This state of affairs is no longer tenable. A profession must have a scientifically defensible body of knowledge to be constantly adjusted and extended. This body of knowledge must be passed on to the next generation of nurses in a descriptive and clear professional language.

The knowledge base necessary to undertake professional nursing must be subject to new ideas and developments, just like the knowledge underlying any other professional activity. Nursing's knowledge base should be constantly assessed in the light of new research. It is, moreover, essential to recognise that the actual content of nursing practice is subject to change which may be initiated by many factors outside nursing itself. Nursing in one country may be very different from nursing in another, and there will be, in addition, many changes over time. The number of nursing specialties is increasing all the time and each specialty is constantly adding to its own body of knowledge. Nurses have to be willing to update their knowledge continuously, and an appreciation of research is essential for this.

Available knowledge is generated by research, and it is the individual enquiring nurse who should and can stimulate such research. The process begins with the asking of questions. Questions test whether the knowledge asked for is available. When somebody asks a question it can either be answered from the existing body of knowledge or not. For example, if the question is: 'Why do we change a patient's position in order to prevent pressure sores?', we can find an answer in the nursing literature. Thus, we can use the answer to justify the practice of changing the patient's position and we can pass this answer on to others.

If we have a question to which we can find no credible answer, that is, there is no available knowledge in the literature, it may be a relevant initial question to spark off research. A person with research experience may have to change the question a little in order to make it researchable, but the essence of the question should be preserved if at all possible. For example, the question 'What is nursing?' is not researchable as it stands; it is a question of policy or ideology rather than research. The questions 'What do nurses do?' or 'What do nurses say about what nursing is?' are researchable. The answer to the first can be obtained by observing nurses and to the second by asking nurses. However, the observing and the asking must follow strict rules, rules which ensure that the results, the data, can be relied on, that they are not too biased. The rules which are followed are part of the research process which has to be learned just as the nursing process has to be learned.

The answers, referred to as research findings, must be fed back into the available body of knowledge, that is, into the literature. Unless research findings are published, they make no contribution to knowledge at all. It is only through published findings that the body of available knowledge can grow.

Different levels of research awareness and competence are required. Firstly, the questions, the importance of which has already been stressed, need to be asked. The wish to question rather than to accept conventional practice, the intellectual curiosity which prompts it, should be an essential quality of all nurses claiming to be professionals. Secondly, with the questions must come the willingness to read professional literature to look for an answer. Answers to the initial questions should be sought by the questioner in the first instance. Whilst we fully recognise the difficulties inherent in keeping up to date with the reading of the rapidly proliferating literature, we also emphasise the need for it. Colleges of nursing and midwifery usually make their library facilities available to qualified nurses in their area and their librarians are more than willing to give help and advice.

Research findings are often presented in a form which cannot easily be interpreted by someone without some basic knowledge of research methods. Their scientific credibility and potential for use must therefore be assessed, and the person making the assessment must have the necessary skill and competence. The profession needs an increasing number of members who have acquired sufficient knowledge in research to help uninitiated colleagues. There are now many possibilities for basic research training. Moreover, many undergraduate and post-basic professional nursing courses include a substantial amount of research methodology and elementary statistics and a small but growing number of courses at Master's level also exist.

In order to initiate research activity and to be responsible for its successful execution, the profession needs people with some advanced knowledge. These research-proficient individuals need not take the research over to the exclusion of everyone else; they can be, and usually are, advisers and leaders of projects. They will, probably, have acquired their expertise on advanced academic courses and through gaining experience as helpers with on-going research.

The need to increase the profession's research commitment is urgent for at least three main reasons. Firstly, research has the potential to initiate helpful changes in the care of patients and clients. If we are to give more than lip service to our quest for excellence in nursing, we require research. Secondly, the economic restraints which pervade most countries make it essential for the profession to support its claims for resources. Cost-effectiveness is demanded, and cost-effectiveness in nursing should be the profession's challenge. Thirdly, professional nursing requires not only a defensible body of knowledge which it can communicate to the next generation of nurses, but it also needs such knowledge for effective interdisciplinary partnership as the basis for shared care.

Nursing needs to defend its activities and this requires research. The responsibility for an increased research commitment must not be left to a few; it must be everybody's concern, and everybody has an important part to play. It is a responsibility which brings excitement and intellectual stimulation. Research awareness, as an attitude to all nursing activities in whatever field, ensures on-going interest and wonder. It can cancel out any feelings of boredom caused by repetitiveness. Active involvement in research brings, in addition to excitement and intellectual stimulation, enormous challenges and surprises. Some inevitable frustrations are easily balanced by experiences of successes and achievements.

All professional groups in the nursing profession have a responsibility to activate the spiral of knowledge (Figure 15.1). Its dynamic nature must not just be preserved but accelerated. The key lies in research, but research can only act as an influential change agent if everyone contributes. Educators must incorporate it into their teaching; administrators must facilitate its process and the use of findings; clinical practitioners must continue to ask questions and use available answers responsibly. The growth and utilisation of available knowledge through research can only be achieved by thoughtful teamwork.

It is our contention that the prospects for a truly research-minded nursing profession are bright. We are equally convinced

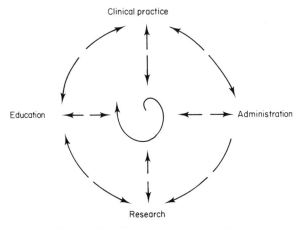

Figure 15.1 The spiral of knowledge

that ignoring/negating our research responsibilities will mean professional suicide. We hope that this small book will make a contribution to the creation of the kind of professional ethos which is based on the dignity of defensible knowledge.

References

Abbey J.C. *et al.* (1978) How long is that thermometer accurate? *American Journal of Nursing*, **78**, 8, 1375–1378

Abdellah F. & Levine E. (1957) Developing a measure of patient and personal satisfaction with nursing care. *Nursing Research*, **5**, 3, 100–108

Adams, G.F. & McIlwraith P.L. (1963) *Geriatric Nursing*. Oxford: Oxford University Press

Adams, M.E., Armstrong-Esther C., Bryar R., Duberley J., Strong G. & Ward E. (1981) Trial run – the nursing process in midwifery. *Nursing Mirror* **153**, 15, 32–35

Alaszewski A. (1986) *Institutional Care and the Mentally Handicapped – The Mental Handicap Hospital*. London: Croom Helm

Allan E. & Goodbody L. (1984) Staff pay hardly any attention to mentally handicapped patients. *Nursing Mirror*, **158**, 17, 10

Allen D. & Donovan T. (1986) The AWS from a parent's point of view: Part 2 – Services' use and consumer satisfaction. *Mental Handicap*, **14**, 2, 71–74

Altschul A. (1972) *Patient-Nurse Interaction: a Study of Interaction Patterns in Acute Psychiatric Wards*. Edinburgh: Churchill Livingstone

ANA (1979a) *Standards for Nursing Practice*. Kansas City: American Nurses Association

ANA (1979b) *Outcome Standards for Cancer Nursing Practice*. Oncology Nursing Society & ANA Division on Medical Surgical Nursing Practice. Kansas City: American Nurses Association

Angerami E. (1980) Epidemiological study of a body temperature in patients in a teaching hospital. *International Journal of Nursing Studies*, **17**, 91–99

Applegate W.B., Akins D., Vanderzwaag R., Thoni K. & Baker M.G. (1983) A geriatric rehabilitation and assessment unit in a community hospital. *Journal of the American Geriatric Society*, **31**, 4, 206–210

Arnott N. (1833) *Elements of Physics or Natural Philosophy*, Vol. 1. London: Longman, Rees, Orme, Brown and Green

Ashworth P. (1980) *Time to Care*. London: Royal College of Nursing

Ashworth P. (1980) *Care to Communicate*. London: Royal College of Nursing

Auld M. (1967) An investigation into the recruitment and integration of nursing staff in hospitals. *International Journal of Nursing Studies*, **4**, 119–169

Auld M. (1976) *How Many Nurses: A Method of Estimating the Requisite Nursing Establishment for a Hospital*. London: Royal College of Nursing

Ayer S. (1984a) Community care: Failure of professionals to meet family needs. *Child: Care, Health and Development*, **10**, 127–140

Ayer, S. (1984b) Handicapped children in the community. *Nursing Times* Occasional paper, **80**, 117, 66–69

Ayer S. & Alaszewski A. (1984) *Community Care and the Mentally Handicapped: Services for Mothers and their Mentally Handicapped Children*. London: Croom Helm

Ayrshire and Arran Health Board (1985). *Standards of Nursing Practice*. Ayrshire and Arran Health Board

Baillie-Grohman R.C. (1975) The use of a modified form of repertory grid technique. In Fransella F. and Bannister D. (Eds) *A Manual for Repertory Grid Technique*. London: Academic Press

Baker D. (1978) Attidues of nurses to the care of the elderly. Unpublished PhD thesis, University of Manchester

Baker N. *et al.* (1984) The effect of type of thermometer and length of time inserted on oral temperature measurements of afebrile subjects. *Nursing Research*, **33**, 2, 109–111

Ball J.A. (1981) Effect of present patterns of maternity care on the emotional needs of mothers, Parts 1, 2 and 3. *Midwives Chronicle*, **94**, 150–154, 198–202, 231–233

Ball, J.A. (1983) Moving forward in postnatal care: Some aspects of a research project. *Midwives Chronicle*, **93** (Suppl.) 14–16

Ball J.A., Goldstone L.A. & Collier M.M. (1983) *Criteria for Care: The Manual of the North West Nurse Staffing Levels Project*. Newcastle upon Tyne: Polytechnic Products Ltd

Barnet D. & Wainwright P. (1987) A measure of quality. *Senior Nurse*, **6**, 3, 8–9

Barr A., Moores B. & Rhys Hearn C. (1973) A review of the various methods of measuring the dependency of patients on nursing staff. *International Journal of Nursing Studies*, **10**, 195–208

Barton A.A. (1976) The pathogenesis of skin wounds due to pressure.

In Kenedi R.M., Cowden J.M. and Scales J.T. (Eds) *Bed Sore Biomechanics*. London: Macmillan

Barton E.S., Walton J. & Rowe D. (1976) Using grid technique with the mentally handicapped. In Slater P. (Ed.) *Explorations of Personal Space*, Vol. 1. Chichester: John Wiley & Sons

Beail N. (1985) The nature of interactions between nursing staff and profoundly multiply handicapped children. *Child Care, Health and Development*, **11**, 3, 113–129

Beazley J.M. & Ward J.P. (1978) Perineal pain after epidural analgesia in labour. *Midwives Chronicle*, **91**, 204–206

Bergman R. (1987) Research in community nursing. In Littlewood J. (Ed.) *Community Nursing. Recent Advances in Nursing*. Edinburgh: Churchill Livingstone

Black P.M. (1984) Who stops smoking in pregnancy? *Nursing Times*, **80**, 19, 59–61

Black T., Booth K. & Faulkner A. (1984) Co-operation or conflict? How midwives and health visitors view each other's contribution to antenatal education. *Senior Nurse*, **1**, 25–26

Blackwell M.W. (1979) *Care of the Mentally Retarded*. Boston: Little, Brown & Co

Bliss M.R. (1964) A consideration of mechanical methods of preventing bedsores in elderly patients. *Gerontology Clinics*, **6**, 10–21

Bliss M.R., McLaren R. & Exton-Smith A.N. (1966) Mattresses for preventing pressure sores in geriatric patients. *Monthly Bulletin of the Ministry of Health and the Public Health Laboratory Service*, **25**, 238–268

Bloch D. (1977) Criteria, standards, norms, clinical terms in quality assurance. *Journal of Nursing Administration*, **7**, 20–30

Bogdan R. & Taylor S. (1975) This is their home. In Bogdan R. & Taylor S. (Eds) *Introduction to Qualitative Research Methods*. Chichester: John Wiley & Sons

Bogdan R., Taylor S., De Grandpre B. & Haynes S. (1974) Let them eat programs: Attendants' perspectives and programming in wards in state schools. *Journal of Health and Social Behaviour*, **15**, 142–151

Bond S. (1983) Nurses' communication with cancer patients: In Wilson-Barnett J. (Ed.) *Nursing Research, Ten Studies in Patient Care*. Chichester: John Wiley & Sons

Boswell J. (1979) Are classes 4 and 5 paying attention? *Nursing Mirror*, **148**, 12, 24–25

Bowers J. (1984) Is the six week postnatal examination necessary? *The Practitioner*, **229**, 1113–1115

Bowlby J. (1951) *Maternal Care and Mental Health*. Geneva: World Health Organisation

Brain D.T. & Maclay I. (1968) Controlled study of mothers and children in hospital. *British Medical Journal*, **1**, 603–608

Brammer A.C. (1977) *Organised Classes for Pregnant Women and their Partners in Preparation for Childbirth and Parenthood*. An enquiry into the classes provided by the Maternity Services in England in 1975. Maws Ed. Research Scholarship 1974/75. London: Royal College of Midwives

Brockway L. (1986) Hair colour and problems in breast feeding. *Midwives Chronicle*, **99**, 66–67

Brooker C. & Brown M. (1986) National follow-up survey of practising nurse therapists. In Brooking J.I. (Ed.) *Psychiatric Nursing Research*. Chichester: John Wiley & Sons

Brooking J.I. (1985) Advanced psychiatric nursing education in Britain. *Journal of Advanced Nursing*, **10**, 455–468

Brooking J.I. (Ed.) (1986) *Psychiatric Nursing Research*. Chichester: John Wiley & Sons

Brooking J.I. & Minghella E. (1987) Parasuicide. *Nursing Times*, **83**, 21, 40–43

Brown A.J. (1985) School age children with diabetes: knowledge and management of the disease and adequacy of self-concept. *Maternal Child Health Journal*, **14**, 1, 47–61

Brown M.M., Boosinger J., Black J. & Gaspar T. (1985) Nursing innovation for prevention of decubitus ulcers in long term care facilities. *Plastic Surgical Nursing*, **5**, 2, 57–64

Bryar R. (1985) An assessment of the introduction of systematic individualised care into midwives practice. Paper presented to the RCN Research Society Conference 1985

Bryar R. & Strong G. (1983) Trial run – continued. *Nursing Mirror*, **157**, 15, 45–48

Butler R.C. (1985) Towards an understanding of children's difficulties. In Beail N. (Ed.) *Repertory Grid Techniques and Personal Constructs. Applications in Clinical and Educational Settings*. London: Croom Helm

Cahoon M. (Ed.) (1987) *Recent Advances in Nursing – Research Methodology*. Edinburgh: Churchill Livingstone

Callis P.M. (1984) The testing and comparison of the intra-uterine sound against other methods for calming babies. *Midwives Chronicle*, **97**, 336–338

The Campaign for People with Mental Handicaps (1981) *The Principle of Normalisation: A Foundation for Effective Services*. (Available from CMH, 12a Madox Street, London, W1R 9PL.)

Carter J., Hilliard M., Castles M., Stoll L. & Cowan A. (1976) *Standards of Nursing Care: A Guide for Evaluation*. 2nd Edition. London: Springer

Cartwright A. (1964) *Human Relations and Hospital Care*. London: Routledge and Kegan Paul

City and Hackney H.A. (1987) *Achievable Standards of Care for the Elderly Cared for in the Acute Assessment Wards, the Continuing Care Wards, Nursing Homes and Day Hospitals within the City and Hackney H.A.* London: City and Hackney H.A.

Clark J. (1973) *A Family Visitor: A Descriptive Analysis of Health Visiting in Berkshire*. London: Royal College of Nursing

Clark J. (1981) *What do Health Visitors do? A Review of the Research 1960–1980*. London: Royal College of Nursing

Clark J. & Redfern S. (1978) Absence and wastage in nursing. Nursing Times Occasional Paper in two parts. *Nursing Times*, **74**, 11 and 12

Cleland C.C. (1975) *The Profoundly Mentally Retarded*. Englewood Cliffs, New Jersey: Prentice-Hall

Closs J. (1987) Oral temperature measurement. *Nursing Times*, **7**, 36–39

Closs S.J., Macdonald I.A. & Hawthorn P.J. (1986) Factors affecting perioperative body temperature. *Journal of Advanced Nursing*, **11**, 739–744

Conceicao S., Ward M.K. & Kerr D.N.S. (1976) Defects in sphygmomanometers: An important source of error in blood pressure recording. *British Medical Journal*, **1**, 886–888

Consumers Association (1980) *Children in Hospital*. London: Consumers Association

Cook T.D. & Campbell D.T. (1979) *Quasi-experimental Designs and Analysis Issues for Research*. Chicago: Rand MacNally

Cormack D. (1976) *Psychiatric Nursing Observed*. London: Royal College of Nursing

Cormack D. (1984) *The Research Process in Nursing*. Oxford: Blackwell Scientific Publishers

Cormack D.F. (1983) *Psychiatric Nursing Described*. Edinburgh: Churchill Livingstone

Cullen C., Burton M., Watts S. & Thomas M. (1983) A preliminary report on the nature of interactions in a mental handicap institution. *Behaviour Research and Therapy*, **21**, 5, 579–583

CURN Project (1980) *Pre-Operative Sensory Preparation to Promote Recovery*. New York: Grune and Stratton

Daechsel D. & Conine T. A. (1985) Special mattresses: effectiveness in preventing decubitus ulcers in chronic neurologic patients. *Archives of Physical Medicine and Rehabilitation*, **66**, 246–248

Dale J. (1984) Legwork. *Nursing Mirror*, **159**, 20, 22–25

David J. (1984) Clinical forum – tissue breakdown. *Nursing Mirror*, **158**, 10

164   FURTHER RESEARCH FOR NURSING

David J. & Pritchard P. (1987) Using Monitor. *Senior Nurse*, **6**, 4, 42–45

Davies A.D.M. & Peters M. (1983) Stresses of hospitalisation in the elderly; nurses and patients perceptions. *Journal of Advanced Nursing*, **8**, 99–105

Davies C. (1980) *Rewriting Nursing History*. Beckenham: Croom Helm

Davis B. (1984) *Pre-operative Information Giving and Patients' Post-operative Outcome: An Implementation Study*. Report for SHHD. Nursing Studies Unit, University of Edinburgh

Davis B.D. (1986) The strain of training: being a student psychiatric nurse. In Brooking J.I. (Ed.) *Psychiatric Nursing Research*. Chichester: John Wiley & Sons

Dawson J. (1987) Evaluation of a community-based night sitter service. In Fielding P. (Ed.) *Research in the Nursing Care of Elderly People*. Chichester: John Wiley & Sons

Department of Health and Social Security, Scottish Home and Health Department and Welsh Office (1972) *Report of the Committee on Nursing*, p. 130. Cmnd 5115. London: HMSO

Department of Health and Social Security/MAPLIN (1981) Extracts from *Wessex Strategic Planning User Manual*. Manpower Planning Department. Wessex Regional Health Authority MAPLIN Paper 81/13. London: HMSO

Department of Health and Social Security/Operational Research Service (1982) *ORS National Supply Model for Nurses: Review of the Model and Possible Areas for Further Work*. ORS/NURSDI. London: HMSO

Department of Health and Social Security/Operational Research Service (1983) *Nurse Manpower Planning: Approaches and Techniques*. London: HMSO

Department of Health and Social Security (1983) *The Griffiths Report*. London: HMSO

Department of Health and Social Security (1986) *Neighbourhood Nursing – A Focus for Care. Report of the Community Nursing Review* (Chairman: J. Cumerlege). London: HMSO

Dinsdale S.M. (1973) Decubitus ulcers in swine: light and electron microscopy study of pathogenesis. *Archives of Physical Medicine and Rehabilitation*, **54**, 51–56

Donabedian A. (1980) *Explorations in Quality Assessment and Monitoring. Part 1. The Definition of Quality and Approaches to its Assessment*. Health Administration Press. Kansas City: University of Michigan

Donovan I. & Allen D. (1986) The AWS from a parent's point of view: Part I – Attitudes towards integrated services. *Mental Handicap*, **14**, 1, 19–21

Dracup K., Meleis A.I., Clark S., Clyburn A. & Stanley M. (1984) Group counselling in cardiac rehabilitation: effect on patient compliance. *Patient Education and Counselling*, **6**, 4, 169–177

Drayton S. & Rees C. (1984) 'They know what they're doing': The midwife and enemas. *Nursing Mirror*, **159** (5, Suppl.) iv–viii

Duncan A. (1986) Quality assurance in the United Kingdom. In Selbmani H. and Uterla K. (eds). *Quality Assessment of Medical Care*. For Robert Bosch, Stiftung GrübH, by Bleicher Verlag

Dunne L. (1986) Defining quality assurance. *Professional Nurse*, **2**, 47–49

Dunnell K. & Dobbs J. (1982) *Nurses Working in the Community: A Survey Carried out on Behalf of the DHSS in 1980*. London: HMSO

Durham M.L., Swanson B. & Paulford N. (1986) Effect of tachypnoea on oral temperature estimation: a replication. *Nursing Research*, **35**, 4, 211–214

Erickson R. (1980) Oral temperature differences in relation to thermometer and technique. *Nursing Research*, **29**, 3, 157–164

Etheridge P. & Packard R. (1976) An innovative approach to measurement of quality through utilisation of nursing care plans. *Journal of Nursing Administration*, **6**, 42–48

Eusanio P.L. (1976) Monitoring skin care eliminates decubitus ulcers. *American Health Care Association Journal*, 1976, 50–51

Evans G., Beyer S., Todd S. & Blunden R. (1986) Planning for the All Wales Strategy. *Mental Handicap*, **14**, 3, 108–110

Exton-Smith A.N. & Sherwin R.W. (1961) The prevention of pressure sores – significance of spontaneous bodily movements. *Lancet*, **ii**, 1124–1126

Exton-Smith A.N., Wedgwood J., Overstall P.W. & Wallace G. (1982) Use of the 'Air Wave System' to prevent pressure sores in hospital, *Lancet*, **i**, 1288–1290

Fairhurst E. (1978) *Talk and the Elderly in Institutions*. Paper presented to the Annual Conference of Social and Behavioural Gerontology, September 14–16 1978, Edinburgh

Faulkner A. (1979) Monitoring nurse–patient conversation on a ward. *Nursing Times* Occasional Papers, **75**, 23, 95–96

Fawcett J. & Downs F.S. (1986) *The Relationship of Theory and Research*. Connecticut: Appleton Century Crofts

Felce D., Mair T., de Kock U., Saxby H. & Repp A. (1985) An ecological comparison of small community based houses and traditional institutions – II. Physical setting and the use of opportunities. *Behaviour Research and Therapy*, **23**, 3, 337–348

Fenton J., Hartwell C., Jambaccus A., Lee S., Lees J., O'Neill P., Rainford D.J., Rawlinson K., Sweeney B. & Ward J. (1985)

Length of stay in hospital after delivery of a first baby. *Midwives Chronicle*, **98**, 156–159

Field P.A. & Morse J.M. (1985) *Nursing Research. The Application of Qualitative Approaches*. Beckenham: Croom Helm

Fielding P. (1986) *Attitudes Revisited*. London: Royal College of Nursing

Fielding P. (1987) *Research in the Nursing Care of Elderly People*. Chichester: John Wiley & Sons

Flanagan J.C. (1954) The critical incident technique. *Psychological Bulletin*, **51**, 4, 327–358

Forgan Morle K.M. (1984) Patient satisfaction: care of the elderly. *Journal of Advanced Nursing*, **9**, 71–76

Frame S., Moore J., Peters A. & Hall D. (1985) Maternal height and shoe size as predictors of pelvic disproportion: An assessment. *British Journal of Obstetrics and Gynaecology*, **92**, 1239–1245

Garcia J., Garforth S. & Ayres S. (1986) *The Policy and Practice in Midwifery Study: Progress Report*. MIDIRS Information Pack No. 2

Garcia J., Corry M., MacDonald D., Elbourne D. & Grant A. (1984) Mothers' view of continuous electronic fetal heart monitoring and intermittent auscultation in a randomized controlled trial. *Research and the Midwife Conference Proceedings*, 51–67

Garfield S.L. & Bergin A.E. (Eds) (1986) *Handbook of Psychotherapy and Behaviour Change*, 3rd Edn. New York: John Wiley & Sons

Gillett J. (1976) A report on the survey on preparation for childbirth within the catchment area of Copthorne Maternity Unit, Shrewsbury; December 1972–June 1973. *International Journal of Nursing Studies*, **13**, 25–46

Gilmore M. *et al.* (1974) *The Work of the Nursing Team in General Practice*. London: Council for the Education and Training of Health Visitors

Ginsberg G., Marks I. & Waters H. (1985) A controlled cost–benefit analysis. In Marks I. (Ed.) *Psychiatric Nurse Therapists in Primary Care*. London: Royal College of Nursing

Giovannetti P. *et al.* (1986) Measuring quality of nursing care: analysis of reliability and validity of selected instruments. Unpublished report. Alberta: Faculty of Nursing, University of Alberta

Glaser B.G. & Strauss A.L. (1964) Awareness contexts and social interaction. *American Sociological Review*, **29**, 679–699.

Gloucester Area Health Authority (1982) *Total Care Dependency Study at Cheltenham General Hospital*. Unpublished Reports 1 and 2.

Goddard A.A. (1963) *Work Measurement as a Basis for Calculating Nursing Establishments*. Leeds: Leeds Regional Hospital Board

Golden J. (1980) Midwifery training. The views of newly qualified midwives. *Midwives Chronicle*, **93**, 190–194

Goldstone L.A., Ball J.A. & Collier M.M. (1983) *Monitor: An Index of Nursing Care in Medical and Surgical Wards*. Newcastle upon Tyne: Polytechnic Products Ltd

Gordon V. (1986) Reducing depression in women: research in the USA and GB. In Brooking J.I. (Ed.) *Psychiatric Nursing Research*. Chichester: John Wiley & Sons

Gournaky K. (1986) A pilot study of nurses' attitudes with relation to post-basic training. In Brooking J.I. (Ed.) *Psychiatric Nursing Research*. Chichester: John Wiley & Sons

Grant G. (1985) Towards participation in the All Wales Strategy: Issues and processes. *Mental Handicap*, **13**, 2, 51–54

Grant N. (1979) *Time to Care: A Method of Calculating Nursing Workload Based on Individualised Patient Care*. London: Royal College of Nursing

Gregor F.M. (1981) Teaching the patient with ischaemic heart disease – a systematic approach to instructional design. *Patient Counselling and Health Education*, **3**, 2, 57–62

Griffiths R. & Hare M.J. (1985) Do women really want natural childbirth? *Midwives Chronicle*, **98**, 92–94

Groth K.E. (1942) Klinishe beobachtungen und experimentelle studien uber die Enstehung des Dekubitus. *Acta Chirurgica Scandinavica*, **76**, 126–200

Hamilton Smith, S. (1972) *Nil by Mouth*. London: Royal College of Nursing

Harris P.J. (1986) Children, their parents and hospital. In Muller D.J., Harris P.J. and Wattley L. (Eds) *Nursing Children. Psychology Research and Practice*. London: Harper and Row

Harrison S. (1977) *Families in Stress: A Study of the Long Term Medical Treatment of Children and Parental Stress*. London: Royal College of Nursing

Hawthorn P.J. (1974) *Nurse, I Want My Mummy*. London: Royal College of Nursing

Haynes R.B., Gibson E.S., Hackett B.C., Johnson A.L., Sackett D.L., Taylor D.W. & Roberts R.S. (1976) Improvement of medication compliance in uncontrolled hypertension. *Lancet*, *i*, 1265–1268

Hayward J. (1975) *Information: A Prescription Against Pain*. London: Royal College of Nursing

Henderson C. (1984) Influences and interactions surrounding the midwife's decision to rupture the membranes. *Research and the Midwife Conference Proceedings*, 68–85

Hentinen M. (1979) *The Development of the Self-care Ability of Diabetics: the Design Implementation and Evaluation of an*

168 FURTHER RESEARCH FOR NURSING

Experimental Program of Instruction, pp. 93–94. Helsinki: Saitaanhoidon Vuosikirja

Hibbs P. (1982) Pressure sores: a system of prevention. *Nursing Mirror*, **155**, 5, 25–29

Hilton B.A. (1982) Nurses' performance and interpretation of urine testing and capillary blood glucose monitoring measures. *Journal of Advanced Nursing*, **7**, 509–521

Hockey L. (1966) *Feeling the Pulse: A Study of District Nursing in Six Areas*. London: Queen's Institute of District Nursing

Hockey L. (1970) *Co-operation in Patient Care*. London: Queen's Institute of District Nursing

Hockey L. (1972) *Use or Abuse? A Study of the Enrolled Nurse in the District Nursing Service*. London: Queen's Institute of District Nursing

Hockey L. (1985) *Nursing Research – Mistakes and Misconceptions*. Edinburgh: Churchill Livingstone

Holden U.P. & Woods R. (1982) *Reality Orientation: Psychological Approaches to the Confused Elderly*. London: Churchill Livingstone

Holland W.W. (1983) *Evaluation of Health Care*. Oxford: Oxford Medical Publications

Honess T. (1976) Cognitive complexity and social prediction. *British Journal of Social and Clinical Psychology*, **15**, 23–31

Horn B. & Swain M. (1976) An approach to development of criterion measures for quality health care. In American Nurses Association (Ed.) *Issues in Evaluation Research*. Kansas City: ANA

Houston M.J. (1984) Supporting breast feeding at home. *Midwives Chronicle*, **97**, 42–44

Howard J. & Brooking J. (1987) The career patterns of nursing graduates. *International Journal of Nursing Studies*, **24**, 3, 181–190

Howie R. (1985) Client controlled pain relief in childbirth. *Midwives Chronicle*, **98**, 294

Hunt J. (1985) *Nursing Research. Does it Make a Difference*. Proceedings of Second Open Conference of WENR. London: Royal College of Nursing

Hunter M.A. & Williams D. (1985) Mask wearing in the labour ward. *Midwives Chronicle*, **98**, 12–13

Hutchinson A. *et al.* (1985) *Performance Review in Primary Care: Measuring the Effect of Standard Setting*. Unpublished report. Health Care Research Unit, University of Newcastle upon Tyne

Illsley V. & Goldstone L. (1986) Measuring quality in district nursing. *Nursing Times*, **82**, 38–40

Inman V. (1975) *Towards a Theory of Nursing Care*. London: Royal College of Nursing

Isles J. (1986) An eradication campaign. *Nursing Times*, **82**, 32, 59–62

Jackson M.F. (1984) Geriatric rehabilitation on an acute-care medical unit. *Journal of Advanced Nursing*, **9**, 441–448

Jacquerye A. (1984) Choosing an appropriate method of quality assurance. In Willis L. and Linwood M. (Eds) *Measuring the Quality of Nursing Care*. Edinburgh: Churchill Livingstone

Janes N. (1984) A postscript to nursing. In Bell C. and Roberts H. (Eds) *Social Researching*. London: Routledge and Kegan Paul

Jerrett M. (1978) Report of research activities. Unpublished report. University of Edinburgh, Nursing Studies Department

Jerrett M. & Evans K.E. (1986) Children's pain vocabulary. *Journal of Advanced Nursing*, **11**, 403–408

Johnson J.E. (1983) Preparing patients to cope with stress while hospitalised. In Wilson-Barnett J. (Ed.) *Patient Teaching*. Edinburgh: Churchill Livingstone

Jones D.C. & Van Amelswoort Jones G.M.M. (1986) Communication patterns between nursing staff and the ethnic elderly in a long-term care facility. *Journal of Advanced Nursing*, **11**, 265–272

Jones K. (1985) Wound care in the community. *Journal of District Nursing*, **4**, 1, 4–5

Jordan M.M. & Barbenel J.C. (1983) Pressure sore prevalence. In Barbenel J.C., Forbes C.D. and Lowe G.D.O. (Ed.) *Pressure Sores*. London: Macmillan

Kaplan S. & Greenfield S. (1978) Criteria mapping using logic in the evaluation of processes of care. *Quality Review Bulletin*, **4**, 3–7

Kelly G.A. (1955) *The Psychology of Personal Constructs*, Vols. 1 and 2. New York: Norton

Kerr, J., Giovannetti P. & Buchan J. (1985) Dynamics of quality assurance in nursing: a model for evaluation. In *Proceedings of Second Open Conference of the WENR*. London: Royal College of Nursing

Kirchmeier R. (1984) Influences on mother's reactions to Caesarean birth. *Research and the Midwife Conference Proceedings*, 86–101

Kirkham M.J. (1983) Labouring in the dark: Limitations on the giving of information to enable patients to orientate themselves to the likely events and time scale of labour. In Wilson-Barnett, J. (Ed.) *Nursing Research: Ten Studies in Patient Care*. Chichester: John Wiley & Sons

Kitson A. & Kendall H. (1986) Quality assurance. *Nursing Times*, **82**, 29–31

Klinzing D.R. & Klinzing D.G. (1977) *The Hospitalised Child: Communication Technique for Health Personnel*. Englewood Cliffs, New Jersey: Prentice-Hall

Knights J. (1986) Use of meptazinol in routine obstetric practice in a district hospital. *Midwives Chronicle*, **99**, 182–183

Knudson K.G., Spiegel T.M. & Furst D.E. (1981) Outpatient

educational programme for rheumatoid arthritic patients. *Patient Counselling and Health Education*, **3**, 77–82

Kratz C.R. (1978) *Care of the Long-Term Sick in the Community*. Edinburgh: Churchill Livingstone

Kübler Ross E. (1973) *On Death and Dying*. London: Tavistock Publications

Laidman P. (1987) *The Health Visitor's Role in the Prevention of Accidents to Children between Ante-natal and Pre-school Age*. London: Health Education Authority

Lancour J. (1976) How to avoid pitfalls in measuring blood pressure. *American Journal of Nursing*, **76**, 5, 773–775

Lathlean J. & Farmish S. (1984) *Ward Sister Training Project. Nursing Education Research Unit Report*. London: Kings College, University of London

Le May A.G. & Redfern S.J. (1987) A study of non-verbal communication between nurses and elderly patients. In Fielding P. (Ed). *Research in the Nursing Care of Elderly People*. Chichester: John Wiley & Sons

Lefton E., Bonstelle S. & Frengley J.D. (1983) Success with an inpatient geriatric unit; a controlled study of outcome and follow-up. *Journal of the American Geriatric Society*, **31**, 3, 149–155

Leininger M. (Ed.) (1985) *Qualitative Research Methods in Nursing*. New York: Grune and Stratton

Levine D.M., Green L.W., Deeds S.G., Chwalow J., Russell R.P. & Finlay J. (1979) Health education for hypertensive patients. *Journal of the American Medical Association*, **241**, 1700–1703

Levine P.H. & Britten A.F.H. (1973) *Supervised patient management of haemophilia. Annals of Internal Medicine*, **78**, 195–201

Levy V. (1984) The 'third day blues'. *Midwives Chronicle*, **97** (Suppl.), xiv–xv

Lindeman C. (1975) Delphi survey of priorities in clinical nursing research. *Nursing Research*, **24**, 434–441

Lindheim R., Glaser H.H. & Coffin C. (1972) *Changing Hospital Environments for Children*. Harvard, Mass.: Harvard University Press

Littlewood J. (1987) Community nursing – an overview. In Littlewood J. (Ed.) *Community Nursing. Recent Advances in Nursing*. Edinburgh: Churchill Livingstone

Lowthian P.T. (1970) Bedsores – the missing links? *Nursing Times*, **66**, 46, 1454–1458

Lowthian P.T. (1977) A review of pressure sore prophylaxis. *Nursing Mirror*, **144**, 11 (Suppl.), vii–xv

Lowthian P.T. (1979) Pressure sore prevalence. *Nursing Times*, **75**, 358–360

Lowthian P.T. (1987) The practical assessment of pressure sore risk. *Care Science and Practice*, **5**, 4, 3–7

Luker K. (1981) The role of the health visitor. In Kinniard J. *et al.* Edinburgh: Churchill Livingstone

Luker K.A. (1982) *Evaluating Health Visiting Practice: an Experimental Study to Evaluate the Effects of Focused Health Visiting Intervention on Elderly Women Living Alone at Home*. London: Royal College of Nursing

MacDonald H. (1985) *A Humane and Dignified Task? An Exploratory Study of Nursing in Psychiatric Rehabilitation*. Project submitted for BSc (Hons) Nursing Studies, Chelsea College (copies in the University of London libraries at King's College and St George's Medical School)

McFarlane J. (1970) *The Proper Study of the Nurse*. London: Royal College of Nursing

McFarlane J. (1979) Take aim and shoot for goal. *Nursing Mirror*, **148**, Supplement, xx–xxiv

MacGuire J. (1969) *Threshold to Nursing: A Review of the Literature on Nurse Training Programmes in the U.K.* Occasional Papers in Social Administration No. 30. London: Bell

MacIlwaine H. (1983) The communication patterns of female neurotic patients with nursing staff in psychiatric units of general hospitals. In Wilson-Barnett J. (Ed.) *Nursing Research: Ten Studies in Patient Care*. Chichester: John Wiley & Sons

McIntosh J. (1981) Communicating with patients in their own homes. In Macleod Clark J. and Bridge W. (Eds) *Communication in Nursing Care*. Chichester: John Wiley & Sons

McIntosh J.B. & Richardson I.M. (1976) *Work Study of District Nursing Staff*. Scottish Health Service Studies 37. Edinburgh: SHHD

Maclean D. (1977) An appraisal of the concepts of infant feeding and their application in practice. *Journal of Advanced Nursing*, **2**, 111–126

Macleod Clark J. (1983). An analysis of nurse–patient conversations on surgical wards. In Wilson Barnett J.C. (Ed.) *Nursing Research, Ten Studies in Patient Care*. Chichester: John Wiley & Sons

Macleod Clark J. (1986) In Redfern S.J. (Ed.) *Nursing Elderly People*. Edinburgh: Churchill Livingstone

Macleod Clark J., Kendall S. & Haverty S. (1987) Helping nurses develop their health education role. *Nurse Education Today*, **7**, 63–68

Maggs C. (1981) Control mechanisms and the new nurses, 1881–1914. *Nursing Times* Occasional Paper, **25**, 97–100

Mahaffy P.R. (1965) The effects of hospitalisation on children admitted for tonsillectomy and adenoidectomy. *Nursing Research*, **14**, 12–19

Majesky S., Bresler M. & Nishlo K. (1978) Patient indicators of nursing care. *Nursing Research*, **27**, 365–371

Mancia G. *et al.* (1983) Effects of blood pressure measurements – by the doctor on patient's blood pressure and heart rate. *Lancet*, **2**, 695–698

Mander R. (1983) Stop and consider: Student midwife wastage in training. *Research and the Midwife Conference Proceedings*, 38–52

Marks I.M. (1985) *Psychiatric Nurse Therapists in Primary Care.* London: Royal College of Nursing

Marks I.M., Bird J. & Lindley P. (1978) Psychiatric nurse therapists 1978 – developments and implications. *Behavioural Psychotherapy*, **6**, 25–35

Marks I.M., Connolly J., Hallam R. & Philpott R. (1975) Nurse therapists in behavioural psychotherapy. *British Medical Journal*, **iii**, 144–148

Marks I.M., Connolly J., Hallam R. & Philpott R. (1977) *Nursing in Behavioural Psychotherapy: An Advanced Clinical Role for Nurses.* London: Royal College of Nursing

Mathews A. & Ridgeway V. (1981) Personality and surgical recovery: a review. *British Journal of Clinical Psychology*, **20**, 243–260

Mayou R., MacMahon D., Sleight D. & Florence M.T. (1981) Early rehabilitation after myocardial infarction. *Lancet*, **ii**, 1399–1401

Melia K. (1982) 'Tell it as it is' – qualitative method and nursing research. *Journal of Advanced Nursing*, **7**, 4, 327–336

Melia K.M. & Macmillan M.S. (1983) *Nurses and the Elderly in Hospital and the Community: A Study of Communication.* Edinburgh: Nursing Studies Research Unit, University of Manchester

Melzack R. (1975) The McGill Pain Questionnaire: major properties and scoring methods. *Pain*, **1**, 277–299

Melzack R. & Torgerson W.S. (1971) On the language of pain. *Anaesthesiology*, **34**, 50–59

Mercer G. (1979) *The Employment of Nurses. Nursing Labour Turnover in the NHS.* London: Croom Helm

Merchant M. & Saxby P. (1981) Reality orientation; a way forward. *Nursing Times*, **77**, 33

Methven R. (1982) The antenatal booking interview: Recording an obstetric history or relating to a mother-to-be? *Research and the Midwife Conference Proceedings*, Part 1, 63–76; Part 2, 77–95

Miller A. (1985) A study of the dependency of eldery patients in wards using different methods of nursing care. *Age and Ageing*, **14**, 132–138

Miller A.E. (1978) *Evaluation of the Care Provided for Patients with*

Dementia in Six Hospital Wards. Unpublished MSc thesis, University of Manchester

Ministry of Health (1959) *Report of the Committee on the Welfare of Children in Hospital*. (Chairman: Sir Harry Platt). London: HMSO

Montgomery-Robinson K. (1986) Accounts of health visiting. In White A. (Ed.) *Research in Preventive Community Care*. Chichester: John Wiley & Sons

Moorat D.S. (1976) The cost of taking temperatures. *Nursing Times*, **72**, 767–770

Moores B. & Thompson A. (1986) What 1357 hospital inpatients think about aspects of their stay in British acute hospitals. *Journal of Advanced Nursing*, **11**, 87–102

Moss J.R. (1981) Helping your children to cope with the physical examination. *Paediatric Nursing*, **7**, 17–20

Muir-Cochrane E. (1986) An examination of the psychiatric nursing component of degree/RGN courses in Britain. In Brooking J.I. (Ed.) *Psychiatric Nursing Research*. Chichester: John Wiley & Sons

Munhall P.L. & Oiler C.J. (1986) *Nursing Research – A Qualitative Perspective*. Connecticut: Appleton Century Crofts

Nichols G.A. & Kucha D.H. (1972) Oral measurements. *American Journal of Nursing*, **72**, 6, 1091–1092

Nichols G.A., Ruskin M.M., Glor B.A. *et al.* (1966) Oral, axillary and rectal temperature determinations and relationships. *Nursing Research*, **15**, 307–310

North Eastern Regional Hospital Board, Scotland (1967, 1969) *Nursing Workload as a Basis for Staffing* (Scottish Health Service Studies No. 3 and No. 9). Edinburgh: Scottish Home and Health Department

Northern Regional Health Authority/South Tyneside Area Health Authority (1978) *Report on the Evaluation of the Aberdeen Formula for Calculating Nurse Establishments in Hospital Wards*

Norton D., McLaren R. & Exton-Smith A.N. (1975, reprint). *An Investigation of Geriatric Nursing Problems in Hospital*. Edinburgh: Churchill Livingstone

Notter L.E. (1974) *Essentials of Nursing Research*. New York: Springer-Verlag

Nudds L. (1987) Healing information. *Nursing Times Community Outlook*, September, 12–14

O'Brien E. & O'Malley K. (1981) *Essentials of Blood Pressure Measurement*. Edinburgh: Churchill Livingstone

Open University (1979) *Research Methods in Education and the Social Sciences. Blocks 1–8*. Milton Keynes: Open University Press.

Openshaw S. (1984) Literature review: measurement of adequate care. *International Journal of Nursing Studies*, **21**, 4, 295–304

Orem D. (1980) *Nursing: Concepts of Practice*, 2nd Edn. London: McGraw Hill

Oswin M. (1978) *Children in Long Stay Hospitals*. London: Heinemann/SIMP

Ozbolt Goodwin J. (1979) Programmed instruction for self-care following pulmonary surgery. *International Journal of Nursing Studies*, **16**, 29–40

Padilla G. & Grant M. (1982) Quality assurance programmes for nursing. *Journal of Advanced Nursing*, **7**, 135–145

Paget J. (1873) Clinical lecture on bed-sores. *The Students' Journal and Hospital Gazette*, 1873, 144–146

Parnell J.W. (1978) *Community Psychiatric Nursing: a Descriptive Study*. London: Queen's Nursing Institute

Partridge J., Chisholm N. & Levy B. (1985) Generalisation and maintenance of ward programmes: Some thoughts on organisational factors. *Mental Handicap*, **13**, 1, 26–29

Paton X. & Petrusev B. (1974) The stimulation of verbal skills in the high grade mentally retarded patient: a nurse administered treatment procedure. *International Journal of Nursing Studies*, **11**, 2, 119–126

Pattie A.H. & Gilleard C.J. (1979) *CAPE scales. Manual of the Clifton Assessment Procedures for the Elderly*. Essex: Hodder and Stoughton

Paykel E.S. & Griffith J.H. (1983) *Community Psychiatric Nursing for Neurotic Patients*. London: Royal College of Nursing

Pearson A. (Ed.) (1987) *Nursing Quality Measurement. Quality Assurance and Methods for Peer Review*. Chichester: John Wiley & Sons

Phaneuf M. (1976) *The Nursing Audit*. Connecticut: Appleton Century Crofts

Pinkerton P. (1980) Preparing children for surgery. *On Call*, 5th June, 8–9

Polit D. & Hungler B. (1983) *Nursing Research Principles and Methods*, 2nd Edition. Philadelphia: Lippincott Co.

Polit D. & Hungler B. (1985) *Essentials of Nursing Research*, 2nd Edition. Philadelphia: Lippincott Co.

Pope V.E. (1986) Midwifery training in Scotland: An opinion survey. *Midwives Chronicle*, **99**, 198–200

Porter C.S. (1974) Grade school children's perceptions of their internal body parts. *Nursing Research*, **23**, 5, 384–391

Poster E.C. (1983) Stress immunisation: Techniques to help children cope with hospitalisation. *Maternal Child Nursing Journal*, **12**, 119–134

Powell D. (1982) *Learning to Relate: A Study of Student Psychiatric Nurses' Views of their Preparation and Training*. London: Royal College of Nursing

Pugh Davies S., Kassab J.Y., Thrush A.J. Smith P.H.S. (1986) A comparison of mercury and digital clinical thermometers. *Journal of Advanced Nursing*, **11**, 535–543

Pullan B. & Chittock J. (1986) Quantifying quality. *Nursing Times*, **82**, 38–39

Rahe R.H., Scalzi C. & Shine K. (1975) A teaching evaluation questionnaire for post-myocardial infarction patients. *Heart Lung*, **4**, 759–766.

Raiman J. (1986) Monitoring pain at home. *Journal of District Nursing*, **4**, 11, 4–6

Raphael W. (1967) Do we know what patients think? A survey comparing the views of patients, staff and committee members. *International Journal of Nursing Studies*, **4**, 209–223

Raphael W. (1969) *Patients and their Hospitals*. London: King Edward's Hospital Fund for London

Raphael W. (1977) *Patients and their Hospitals*. London: King Edward's Fund for London

Raphael W. (1979) *Old People in Hospital*. London: King Edward's Fund

Ravenette A.T. (1975) Grid techniques for children. *Journal of Child Psychology and Psychiatry*, **16**, 79–83

Rawlings S.A. (1985) Life styles of severely retarded non-communicating adults in hospitals and small residential homes. *British Journal of Social Work*, **15**, 281–293

RCGP (1985) *What Sort of Doctor? Assessing Quality of Care in General Practice*. Report from General Practice No. 23. London: RCGP

RCN (1977) *Ethics Related to Research in Nursing*. London: Royal College of Nursing

RCN (1980) *Standards of Nursing Care*. London: Royal College of Nursing

RCN (1981) *Towards Standards*. London: Royal College of Nursing

RCN (1985) *The Education Of Nurses: A New Dispensation*. Commission of Nursing Education. London: Royal College of Nursing

RCN (1987) *Nursing Quality Assurance Directory*. London: Royal College of Nursing

Redfern S. (1986) Maintaining healthy skin. In Redfern S. (Ed.) *Nursing Elderly People*. Edinburgh: Churchill Livingstone

Reed M.A. (In press) Global perspective. In Brooking J.I. (Ed.) *Textbook of Psychiatric Nursing*. Edinburgh: Churchill Livingstone

Reedy B.L.E.C. *et al.* (1976) Nurses and nursing in primary medical care in England. *British Medical Journal*, **2**, 1304–1306

Reedy B.L.E.C. *et al.* (1980) A comparison of activities and opinions of attached and employed nurses in general practice. *Journal of the Royal College of General Practitioners*, **217**, 483–489

Reichel S. (1958) Shearing force as a factor in dedecubitus ulcers in paraplegics. *J. Amer. Med. Assoc.*, **166**, 762

Reid N. & Boore J. (1987) *Research Methods and Statistics in Health Care*, London: Edward Arnold

Revans R. (1964) *Standards for Morale: Cause and Effect in Hospitals.* Nuffield Provincial Hospitals Trust

Rhys-Hearn C. (1977) Nursing workload determination: Development and trials of a package. *Medical Informatics*, **2**, 2

Rhys-Hearn C. & Potts D. (1978) The effects of patients' individual characteristics upon activity times for items of nursing care. *International Journal of Nursing Studies*, **15**, 23–50

Ridgeway V. & Mathews A. (1983) Psychological preparation for surgery. A comparison of methods, *British Journal of Clinical Psychology*, **21**, 271–280

Roberts I. (1975) *Discharged from Hospital.* London: Royal College of Nursing

Robertson J. (1956) A mother's observations on the tonsillectomy of her four year old daughter (with comments by Anna Freud). *The Psychoanalytic Study of the Child*, **11**, 410–433

Robertson J. (1970) *Young Children in Hospital.* London: Tavistock

Robinson S. (1986) Career intentions of newly qualified midwives. *Midwifery*, **2**, 25–36

Robinson S., Golden J. & Bradley S. (1983) *A Study of the Role and Responsibilities of the Midwife. Nursing Education Research Unit Report No. 1.* London: King's College, University of London

Rodin J. (1983) *Will This Hurt? Preparing Children for Hospital and Medical Procedures.* London: Royal College of Nursing

Rogers E.C. (1978) Nursing management in relation to beds used within the national spinal injuries centre for the prevention of pressure sores. *Paraplegia*, **16**, 147–153

Romney M.L. (1980) Predelivery shaving: An unjustified assault? *Journal of Obstetrics and Gynaecology*, **1**, 33–35

Romney M.L. (1983) Chair project. *Research and the Midwife Conference Proceedings*, 69–80

Romney M.L. & Gordon J. (1981) Is your enema really necessary? *British Medical Journal*, **282**, 1269

Ross F.M. (1988) Information sharing between patients, nurses and doctors. In Johnson R. (Ed.) *Excellence in Nursing.* Recent Advances Series. Edinburgh: Churchill Livingstone

Salzer J.E. (1975) Classes to improve diabetic self care. *American Journal of Nursing*, **75**, 1324–1326

Savage B., Widdowson T. & Wright T. (1979) Improving the care of the elderly. In Towell D. & Harries C. (Eds) *Innovation in Patient Care*. London: Croom Helm

Scales J.T., Lowthian P.T., Poole A.G. & Ludman W.R. (1982) 'Vaperm' patient-support system: A new general purpose hospital mattress. *Lancet*, **ii**, 1150–1152

Schröeck R. (1977) *The Ongoing Process of Re-appraisal. An investigation into the Principles of Health Visiting*. London: Council for Education and Training of Health Visitors

Seaman C. & Verhonick P. (1982) *Research Methods for Undergraduate Students in Nursing*, 2nd Edition. New York: Appleton Century Crofts

Sechrist K.R. (1979) The effect of repetitive teaching on patients knowledge about drugs to be taken home. *International Journal of Nursing Studies*, **16**, 51–58

Shaw C. (1986a) *Introducing Quality Assurance*. Kings Fund Project Paper No. 64. London: King's Fund

Shaw C. (1986b) *Quality Assurance: What the Colleges are Doing*. Quality Assurance Project Report, London: Kings Fund

Shaw M. & Heyman B. (1982) Changes in patterns of care of the mentally handicapped: Implications for nurses' perceptions of their roles and hospital decision making processes. *Journal of Advanced Nursing*, **7**, 555–563

Shelley S.I. (1984) *Research Methods in Nursing and Health*. Boston: Little, Brown & Co.

Sims R.S. (1965) Temperature taking in a teaching hospital. *Lancet*, **ii**, 535–536

Sims-Williams A.J. (1976) Temperature taking with glass thermometers: A review. *Journal of Advanced Nursing*, **1**, 481–493

Skeet M. (1970) *Home from Hospital*. London: Dan Mason Nursing Research Committee

Skidmore D. (1986) The effectiveness of community psychiatric nursing teams and base-locations. In Brooking J.I. (Ed.) *Psychiatric Nursing Research*. Chichester: John Wiley & Sons

Sladden S. (1979) *Psychiatric Nursing in the Community: A Study of the Working Situation*. Edinburgh: Churchill Livingstone

Sleep J., Grant A., Garcia J., Elbourne D., Spencer J. & Chalmers I. (1984) West Berkshire perineal management trial. *British Medical Journal*, **289**, 587–590

Smith J. (1981) The idea of health: a philosophical inquiry. *Advances in Nursing Science*, **3**, 43

Smith P. (1984) Towards quality. *Senior Nurse*, **1**, 34, 10–11

Smith P. (1987) The relationship between quality of care and the ward as a learning environment. *Journal of Advanced Nursing*, **12**, 4, 413–421

Spitzer S. (1975) Towards a Marxian theory of deviance. *Social Problems*, **2**, 638–651

Stewart C.P.U. (1980) A prediction score for geriatric rehabilitation prospects. *Rheumatology and Rehabilitation*, **19**, 239–245

Stewart P., Hillan E. & Calder A. (1983) A randomised trial to graduate the use of a birth chair for delivery. *Lancet*, **ii**, 1296–1298

Stockwell F. (1972) *The Unpopular Patient*. London: Royal College of Nursing

Street C.G. (1982) *An Investigation of the Priority on Nurse–Patient Interaction by Psychiatric Nurses*. Project submitted for BSc (Hons) Nursing Studies. Chelsea College (copies in the University of London libraries at King's College and St George's Medical School)

Stronge J.L. & Newton G. (1980) Electronic thermometers – a costly rise in efficiency. *Nursing Mirror*, **151**, 29

Sturmey P., Crisp T. & Dearden B. (1983) Room management with profoundly handicapped young adults. *Mental Handicap*, **11**, 3, 118–119

Takacs K.M. & Valenti W.M. (1982) Temperature measurement in a clinical setting. *Nursing Research*, **31**, 6, 368–370

Tam G. (1979) A comparison of two electronic sphygmomanometers with the traditional mercury type. *Nursing Times*, **75**, 880–885

Taylor T.V., Rimmer S., Day B., Butcher J. & Dymock I.W. (1974) Ascorbic acid supplementation in the treatment of pressuresores. *Lancet*, **ii**, 544–546

Telford W.A. (1979) *Determining Nursing Establishments*. Health Service Manpower Review, Vol. 5, No. 4

Thompson D.R. (1981) Recording patients blood pressure: A review. *Journal of Advanced Nursing*, **6**, 283–290

Thomson A. (1984) Antenatal care: An examination of the midwife's contribution. *Research and the Midwife Conference Proceedings*, 135–162

Tierney A. (1973) Toilet training. *Nursing Times*, **69**, 1740–1745

Tierney A.J. (1983) *Nurses and the Mentally Handicapped*. Chichester: John Wiley & Sons

Torrance C. (1986) The physiology of wound healing. *Nursing*, 3rd series, **3**, 5, 162–168

Towell D. (1975) *Understanding Psychiatric Nursing: A Sociological Study of Modern Psychiatric Nursing Practice*. London: Royal College of Nursing

Towell D. & Harries C. (1979) *Innovation in Patient Care*. London: Croom Helm

Treece E.W. & Treece J.W.Jr (1982) *Elements of Research in Nursing*. St Louis: C. V. Mosby

United Kingdom Central Council for Nursing, Midwifery and Health Visiting (1986) *Project 2000*. London: UKCC

Unwin K. (1981) *A Case Study to Investigate Problems Faced by Nurses on a Psychogeriatric Ward*. Project submitted for BSc (Hons) Nursing Studies, Chelsea College (copies in the University of London libraries at King's College and St George's Medical School)

Van Maanen H. (1979) Perspectives and problems on quality of nursing care: an overview of contributions from North America and recent developments in Europe. *Journal of Advanced Nursing*, **4**, 377–389

Vaughn C.E. & Leff J.P. (1976) The influence of family and social factors on the course of psychiatric illness: a comparison of schizophrenic and depressed neurotic patients. *British Journal of Psychiatry*, **129**, 125–137

Ventura M., Hageman P., Slakter M. & Fox R. (1980) Inter-rater reliabilities for two measures of nursing care quality. *Research in Nursing and Health*, **3**, 25–32

Ventura M., Hageman P., Slakter M. & Fox R. (1982) Correlations of two quality of nursing care measures. *Research in Nursing and Health*, **5**, 37–43

Ventura M.R. & Woligora-Serafin B. (1981) Study priorities identified by nurses in mental health settings. *International Journal of Nursing Studies*, **18**, 41–46

Visintainer M.A. & Wolfer J. A. (1974) Psychological preparation for surgical paediatric patients: the effect on children's and parents' stress responses and adjustment. *Paediatrics*, **56**, 187–202

Wandelt M.A. & Ager J. (1970) *Quality Patient Care Scales (QUAL-PACS)*. Detroit: Wayne State University

Wainwright P. & Burnips S. (1983a) Qualpacs at Burford. *Nursing Times*, **79**, 36–38

Wainwright P. & Burnips S. (1983b) Qualpacs the second visit. *Nursing Times*, **79**, 26–27

Walker J.F. (1976) Midwife or obstetric nurse? Some perceptions of midwives and obstetricians of the role of the midwife. *Journal of Advanced Nursing*, **1**, 129–138

Walker M. (1984) Observation in the newly admitted patient. *Nursing Times*, 29–32

Walker V.H. & Selmanoff E.D. (1965) A note on the accuracy of temperature, pulse and respiration procedure. *Nursing Research*, **14**, 1, 72–76

Watson M. & Morrison E.M. (1979) Health education and infant feeding – does mother know best? *Midwives Chronicle*, **92**, 220–221

Wells T.J. (1980) *Problems in Geriatric Nursing Care*. Edinburgh: Churchill Livingstone

Welsh Office (1985) *Midwifery Sub-group. All Wales Nurse Manpower Planning Group. Standards of Care*. Welsh Office

West Midland Regional Health Authority (1979) *Using the Civil Service Manpower Planning Models on Nurse Staffing Problems*. Management Services Division Operational Research. Birmingham: West Midlands Regional Health Authority

West Midlands Regional Health Authority (1980) *Use of the Trent Nursing Formula*. MAPLIN paper 80/110. London: HMSO

White E. (1986) Factors influencing general practitioners to refer patients to community psychiatric nurses. In Brooking J.I. (Ed.) *Psychiatric Nursing Research*. Chichester: John Wiley & Sons

Wilcox J. (1961) Observer factors in the measurement of blood pressure. *Nursing Research*, **10**, 1, 4–17

Wilkerson V.A. (1984) The use of episiotomy in normal delivery. *Midwives Chronicle*, **97**, 106–110

Williams K. (1974) Ideologies of nursing: their meanings and implications. *Nursing Times*. Occasional paper, **8**, 8, 74

Wilson-Barnett J. (1978) *A Review of Patient Nurse Dependency Studies*. Nursing Research Liaison Group. DHSS

Wilson-Barnett J. (1978) Patients' emotional responses to barium X-rays. *Journal of Advanced Nursing*, **3**, 37–46

Wilson-Barnett J. (1979) *Stress in Hospital: Patients' Psychological Reactions to Illness and Health Care*. Edinburgh: Churchill Livingstone

Wilson-Barnett J. (Ed.) (1983) *Patient Teaching*. Edinburgh: Churchill Livingstone

Wilson-Barnett J. (1984) Alleviating stress for hospitalised patients. *International Review of Applied Psychology*, **33**, 493–503

Wilson-Barnett J. & Oborne J. (1983) Studies of evaluating patient teaching: implications for practice. *Journal of Nursing Studies*, **20**, 1, 33–44

Wood J.R.A. (1985) Room management activity sessions for adults in long stay hospitals: Implications for staff and residents. *Mental Handicap*, **13**, 76–77

Wright D. (1984) An introduction to the evaluation of nursing care: a review of the literature. *Journal of Advanced Nursing Studies*, **9**, 5, 457–467